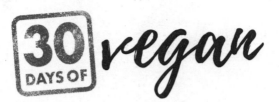

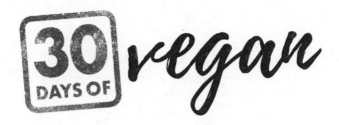

30 DAYS OF vegan

A whole month of
delicious recipes to make
going vegan a breeze

Catherine Kidd R.D.

SEVEN DIALS

First published in Great Britain in 2018 by Seven Dials
An imprint of Orion Publishing Group Ltd
Carmelite House, 50 Victoria Embankment, London, EC4Y 0DZ

An Hachette UK Company

13 5 7 9 10 8 6 4 2

A CIP catalogue record for this book is available
from the British Library.

Paperback ISBN: 9781841882871
Ebook ISBN: 9781841882888

Photography: Vincent Whiteman
Food stylist: Laurie Perry
Prop stylist: Rebecca Newport

Printed and bound by CPI Group (UK) Ltd, Croydon, CR0 4YY

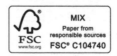

www.orionbooks.co.uk

Contents

Welcome to 30 Days of Vegan!   1
Veganism as a cure: facts vs myths   9
How to eat vegan the right way   17
How to use this book   27
Store cupboard essentials   31

Recipes
Week 1   35
Week 2   77
Week 3   123
Week 4   163
Week 5   201
Snacks   215

Extra Information   228
FAQs about healthy eating   229
Where can I go for more information?   232
References   234
General Index   236
Recipe Index   238
Acknowledgements   241
About the author   242
Cut-out store cupboard essentials   243
Cut-out shopping lists   247
Cut-out menus   257

Welcome to 30 Days of Vegan!

The idea for this book came from two of my friends who wanted to go vegan for Veganuary. They found an almost overwhelming amount of information to help them online, but much of it was misleading or confusing, while many of the recipes they came across were over-complicated. I realised from speaking to my two friends how useful it would be to have a recipe book that could guide people who wanted to try veganism or go vegan for good through the first 30 days, with easy-to-understand and scientifically accurate information. I am a dietitian by trade – I completed a masters in nutrition with a dissertation looking at the effect of vegan diets on the heart and now I work for the NHS and also have my own private practice – so I thought this was something I could put together for them. This book is not saying 'go vegan!' but instead, 'If you're going to go vegan, here's everything you need to make it easy for you, including solid nutrition advice to make sure you do it in the best way.'

Starting any new diet can be daunting, but there is one thing that they all have in common: if it isn't practical and you can't make it fit into your lifestyle, it is doomed to failure from the start. You also need to be able to afford the ingredients required for your particular diet, and be able to find the right foods easily and conveniently, preferably in your local shops. You also need to have the skills to prepare these foods, or know where to buy them ready-prepared when you don't have the time or inclination to cook from scratch.

Hopefully using some of the ideas from this book, as well as the weekly shopping lists and store cupboard essentials lists will make going vegan simple – and enjoyable!

WHY PEOPLE GO VEGAN

First, though, let's look at why people choose to follow a vegan diet. It is an increasingly popular way to eat, but for many different reasons.

1 Animal welfare

Lots of people are worried about the welfare of animals in the meat and dairy industries, and are more and more knowledgeable, interested and concerned about all aspects of their care, from breeding through to husbandry, transportation and their ultimate slaughter. This is likely due to the increased media presence of charities like PETA and the Vegan Society, which both work to highlight the plight of animals and to encourage people to eat a plant-based diet.

2 Environment

The environmental impact of a vegan diet, when compared to that of an omnivorous or vegetarian diet, has been the source of much ongoing debate, research and media attention. At the moment it appears that switching to a vegan diet may be beneficial to the environment in three important areas: carbon footprint, water usage and land usage. But it is worth pointing out that choosing a vegan diet does not automatically make it more environmentally friendly – you also need to consider how your food is grown and processed. For example, some people who eat vegan foods opt for highly processed meat and dairy alternatives such as soya yoghurts and tofu, which have a high environmental impact due to a high carbon footprint during production. Another example is where a high demand for a certain food has resulted in altered land use. For example, our insatiable global appetite for avocados has resulted in mass deforestation and environmental impact.

So in an attempt to make this book as environmentally friendly as possible (although it does have the odd avocado!), I have tried to opt for less-processed foods and attempted to reduce food waste as much as possible, suggesting how to use up any leftovers. I was told recently that in the UK alone, if you stacked up the amount of bread we waste slice for slice, per annum – 24 million slices to be exact – it would be 27 times taller than Mount Everest. That really is staggering, so anything we can do to reduce this and other food waste must be a positive environmental move.

3 Health benefits

Many people go vegan because of the perceived health benefits of a plant-based diet. Despite what the media might say, no diet can cure cancer, reverse the ageing process or wind back the clock on the damage that a poor diet, drinking alcohol and smoking can cause. However, it has been found that vegans do have a lower risk of cardiovascular disease, type 2 diabetes, obesity and some cancers. This is because a vegan diet is often higher in beneficial nutrients (e.g. fibre, magnesium, folic acid, vitamins C and E) and lower in many nutrients implicated in the development of chronic diseases (e.g. calories, saturated fat and cholesterol). For more information on the facts and myths around how veganism can affect your health, see page 9.

Whatever your motivations for going vegan, there are two pros that are both universal and universally appealing . . .

It's cheap

If you compare one omnivorous and one vegan diet of healthy, home-cooked food, the vegan diet is often cheaper. This is because meat and fish can be expensive, especially if you choose to shop for locally sourced, free-range or organic meats, wild fish (rather than farmed) or leaner cuts of meat. It is fair to say that an omnivorous diet of fast foods and refined carbohydrates may be cheaper than buying everything from the shopping lists in this book, but the nutritional content (particularly vitamins and minerals) is in no way comparable.

The most expensive part of a vegan diet is often the collection of herbs and spices you need to add to dishes to make them exciting and different, but you can build up your store cupboard slowly, buying these flavourings as and when you need them. In this book I've included lots of fresh herbs as well as dried, as these add essential colour and taste. If you want to cut down on the cost of a dish, you can switch to dried herbs – the nutritional content won't be affected, but the taste won't be quite the same. Shopping for seasonal fruits and vegetables can make a vegan diet more economical, as well as buying ingredients in bulk, then cooking in large batches to divide up and freeze in portions.

It's easy

Preparing dishes for a home-cooked vegan diet should take no longer than those for an omnivorous diet. This book is designed with busy people in mind; the weekday breakfasts should take no longer than five minutes each to prepare – perfect for people rushing out the door for work – and the lunches and dinners often tie together so that one ingredient can be used in both to save time and money. Cooking in bulk can really help here, too. So if there is a recipe that you particularly like, make more of it and freeze it! If you are going to cook this way, invest in a few small freezerproof containers so that you can freeze each portion separately, otherwise when you come to defrost your food you might not use it all, and you should not re-freeze previously frozen food once thawed, for food safety reasons.

THE PRACTICALITIES OF GOING VEGAN

Once you've thought about why you want to go vegan and have got excited about the pros of this diet, you might want to think about the things you might find tricky, and how you can best work around them. As I said, any diet needs to be practical in order to work, so thinking about the potential challenges isn't something negative, it's sensible.

Eating out

Often this is the greatest challenge for people when they first become vegan. All of us want to eat out every now and again – whether with friends or just because we're on the go. It used to be the case that to eat in cafes or restaurants you would need to go specifically to a vegan outlet to find foods that you would be able to have, but, thankfully, it is becoming increasingly easy to find vegan food now that plant-based eating has become so popular. Now many food items on menus will be marked if they are 'vegan-friendly' and it is even possible to find ready-made sandwiches, salads and snacks at many major high-street food vendors. The Vegan Society has great up-to-date information about where you can look for food when you're 'on the go' (see page 232).

Missing animal products

Whether you miss eating animal products or not will depend on you. One way to combat this is to think about what you can ADD to your diet, rather than what you are taking AWAY. If you think of your pre-vegan food choices and cut out all the animal products, you might be left with just some steamed broccoli and rice. Hardly an exciting meal! So instead think about all the new things you can try to eat more of, such as nuts, seeds, beans, legumes, herbs and spices.

It is easy to buy vegan alternatives of products such as yoghurts, sausages, burgers and cheeses – they are often more processed, but processed food doesn't necessarily mean bad! Sure, you might want to steer clear of lots of added salt and sugar, but do include some of these foods as they are often a great way of adding extra protein to the diet, as they are mainly soya and/or nut based. If you're going vegan for environmental reasons, you may of course opt for fewer of these foods, as the processing may have an adverse environmental impact.

Side-effects

Some people find that going vegan makes them feel bloated and increases flatulence, or you may find you poo more – this is because your diet might be higher in fibre now. Your body is likely to adjust quickly, though, particularly if you previously ate quite a lot of fruits, vegetables and whole grains.

... AND A FEW OTHER IMPORTANT CONSIDERATIONS

If you are serious about cutting out all animal products from your diet, you may find that food shopping initially takes longer when you make the switch to a vegan diet. Lots of foods have 'hidden' animal products in them, so you need to check food labels. For example, gummy sweets often contain gelatin, wineries sometimes use animal products during processing, and many breads contain dairy products such as milk, butter or ghee. Once you get used to label reading, you'll find shopping quicker and easier. Here are a few other things you may be asking yourself:

Is it possible to combine veganism with other diets?

Other diets, such as low FODMAP (see page 14), Paleo, gluten-free or nut allergies, are not catered for in this book. If you don't need to place extra restrictions on your food choices, you shouldn't! If you do need to do so for medical reasons (because you have a diagnosed allergy or are coeliac, for example), seek advice from a dietitian before making extra dietary changes.

Is it safe for children to be vegan?

It is perfectly safe, but it's more challenging to get their diet right! Children are more vulnerable to deficiencies than adults, partly because their fat, protein and vitamin/mineral stores in their bodies are lower, and partly because they need energy to grow rather than just maintain their bodies, unlike adults. This book is not written for children in mind; if you want your child to be vegan, you should speak to a doctor or dietitian who can give you specific, tailored nutritional advice, as a nutritionally inadequate diet can be dangerous for anyone, but particularly so for a growing and developing child.

Where can I find out more information about going vegan?

The Vegan Society has really useful information about different food outlets and supermarkets you can try to source food products, and PETA produces lots of information about Veganuary – so see their websites for more information. However, when it comes to scientific information about the health effects of going vegan, it is always worth speaking to your doctor, dietitian or an Association for Nutrition registered nutritionist, as a lot of the information in the media or on the internet varies between confusing, misleading, and, in some cases, just wrong!

Veganism as a cure: facts vs myths

I've already mentioned that there are health benefits associated with veganism, but that there are also plenty of myths, and as a dietitian, I feel compelled to set the record straight here. So, what does the science really say?

What people say: Vegan diets are good for your heart

Myth or fact: Fact

Risk of cardiovascular disease (heart disease), heart attacks and strokes in vegans is lower than in the rest of the population. This may be because vegans generally have a lower Body Mass Index (BMI), a measure of body weight for height, which is a risk factor for cardiovascular disease when it is high. They generally also have lower blood pressure (this may be because they have a lower BMI) and lower LDL (bad) cholesterol. Vegans, compared with omnivores, consume more fruit and vegetables, which are rich in fibre, folic acid, antioxidants and phytochemicals, all of which are associated with lower cholesterol. Whole grains, soya and nuts all have a protective effect on the heart, and are eaten in greater amounts by vegans than omnivores. Some studies have found vegans are also less likely to smoke tobacco or drink alcohol heavily – habits which also damage your heart health. There are many ways to improve your heart health beyond diet, such as changing your exercise, sleep or stress habits. But changing to a vegan diet may also be of help.

What people say: Following a vegan diet can reduce your risk of cancer

Myth or fact: It's complicated

No diet can cure cancer (despite what the media might say!) and if you are diagnosed with cancer you should seek a medical opinion from a dietitian or doctor before making any changes to your diet. However, choosing a vegan diet may reduce your risk of developing some cancers, such as prostate and bowel cancer. This may be because vegans eat significantly more legumes (a certain family of plant that includes peas, beans, chickpeas and lentils), fruits and vegetables, tomatoes, allium vegetables (such as onions and leeks), fibre and vitamin C than omnivores – and all these foods and nutrients have been found to be protective against these cancers. Red meat and processed meat in particular are linked to an increase risk of colorectal cancer, as well as oesophageal, liver and lung cancers, so by reducing your intake of these foods you can potentially lower your risk. High intake of isoflavone-containing soya products (e.g. soya milk, yoghurt and tofu) in childhood and adolescence has been shown to reduce breast cancer risk in women and prostate cancer risk in men and women in later life. We are still early on in understanding how cancer and diet are linked, and more studies need to be conducted before we can be conclusive about the effect that veganism has on developing the disease and disease progression. If you want to reduce your risk of cancer, following a vegan diet might help, but you could also try a healthy omnivorous diet that is high in fruits, vegetables and soya products and low in red and processed meats.

What people say: Vegan diets help control diabetes

Myth or fact: It's complicated

This is a relatively new area of science, actually – and one that is causing much debate! There are two types of diabetes – 1 and 2. Type 1 refers to the reduced ability of the pancreas to make insulin, while type 2 refers to the reduced ability of the body to respond to the insulin. Insulin is required for all the cells of your body to take up sugar to use for energy, so a lack of insulin means that the sugar level in your blood rises because it cannot get to the cells that need it. Type 1 requires regular injections of insulin and a diet cannot affect the synthesis of insulin, so 'going vegan' will not help. However, there is some evidence that a vegan diet can help with blood sugar control in type 2 diabetes. There are certain nutrients we know to help with type 2 diabetes control – including whole grains, cereals and legumes – so if you follow a vegan diet high in these foods you may improve your glycaemic control. We also know that alcohol, exercise and body fat (among other things!) affect your blood sugar control in type 2 diabetes, so these are definitely areas of your lifestyle you should take control of if you are diagnosed with this type of diabetes.

Always seek professional advice from your doctor or dietitian when making dietary changes if you are diagnosed with diabetes.

What people say: Vegan diets are bad for bone health

Myth or fact: Myth

The vegan diet excludes dairy, which is a great source of calcium. Calcium is a really important nutrient for the body as it is essential for bone health. Bone density builds up during childhood and peaks around puberty, before declining. This rate of decline is faster for women than for men, so making sure you have lots of calcium when you are younger is crucial for building up maximum bone density. Women and children particularly need to focus on getting sufficient calcium in their diet, as well as people who are breastfeeding, women past the menopause, people with coeliac disease, osteoporosis and inflammatory bowel disease.

While a poorly balanced vegan diet is bad for your bones, so too is an unbalanced omnivorous diet. Vegans generally have a lower intake of calcium per day compared to omnivores, which could affect how easily bones fracture, but there are ways to ensure you get enough calcium on a vegan diet (see 'Calcium-rich foods' on page 22). When you 'go vegan', make sure you have lots of these calcium-rich foods and your bones won't suffer.

What people say: Going vegan helps you lose weight

Myth or fact: It's complicated

People lose weight when the number of calories taken in are fewer than calories out. Calories are a measure of energy, and they are contained within carbohydrates, proteins and fats. Calories in simply means the ones you eat, whereas calories out are the ones you burn up through exercise and just keeping your body functioning every day. So if you go on a vegan diet and you use up more calories than you eat, you will lose weight.

That said, many people who switch to a vegan diet DO lose weight. This could be for a number of reasons, the main one being that on a vegan diet you cut out many sources of fat, such as meat and dairy. Another reason is that it's harder to buy vegan food when you're out and about, so it's not so easy to snack. Because of this, if you want to lose weight then going vegan could be an option for you. My main advice, however, is to make sure following this diet is sustainable. It is much more beneficial for health and weight loss to avoid 'yo-yo' dieting by adopting healthy, consistent, new food habits – so don't go vegan as a short-term solution for your waistline. It is essential to make sure you still have adequate nutrition (calories, protein, carbohydrate, fats, vitamins and minerals) and don't lose weight too quickly as this can be damaging to your body and cause you to gain weight easily in the future.

If you want to adopt a vegan lifestyle but do not want to lose weight, that's OK, too. By including plenty of healthy fats, such as nuts and seeds, you can maintain your current weight. If you find yourself losing weight without wanting to, try some of the dairy alternatives that are high in calories, such as coconut yoghurt. This book has calorie counts in it, to make sure your body is getting enough energy. The average woman should aim for 2000 calories per day for healthy weight and body maintenance, while the average man should be aiming for 2500 (more if you're very active).

What people say: Going vegan makes you iron deficient

Myth or fact: Myth

There are two types of iron: heme and non-heme. Heme iron is found in red meat and is the more easily absorbed form. Non-heme iron is found in fruits and vegetables; it is less easily absorbed, but having a diet high in vitamin C helps you to absorb it. Therefore, although vegans have more of the iron that is hard to absorb and less of the iron that is easy to absorb, the rates of iron deficiency anaemia between vegans and omnivores isn't that different. If you feel tired all the time, look pale, have shortness of breath or heart palpitations, they could be signs of iron deficiency anaemia, so you should check your iron levels with your GP.

What people say: Veganism helps if you have Irritable Bowel Syndrome (IBS)

Myth or fact: Myth

The vegan diet is very high in short chain carbohydrates known as FODMAPs. These molecules can actually increase IBS symptoms, so limiting them can help reduce symptoms. There is one diet, called the low FODMAP diet, which is evidence-based and advocates reducing your intake of these specific carbohydrates (FODMAPs) to help improve IBS symptoms. It is a diet that is highly restrictive, especially when you start off and before you can begin to reintroduce foods into your diet. There is no evidence that a vegan diet could improve your IBS symptoms, and combining two restrictive diets, such as veganism and the low FODMAP diet, could be dangerous for your health as you will limit many essential nutrients in your diet. If you suffer from Irritable Bowel Syndrome, you must ask to be referred to a specialist dietitian for advice on the low FODMAP diet before trying it out alone.

What people say: Veganism is good for mental health

Myth or fact: It's complicated – all healthy food helps!

Some people say eating less meat improves their mood, but there is no actual evidence that a vegan diet *per se* is good for your mental health. Food can affect your mood in two different ways. By having quality carbohydrates, healthy fats, staying hydrated and limiting alcohol consumption, your mood is likely to be improved. This is all part of a balanced diet and having regular meals. Secondly, your relationship with food can affect your mood. If going vegan helps you improve the balance in your diet – focusing on healthy fats and good carbohydrates – it could, in theory, help your mood, but this is very much unproven. Mental health can be affected by many lifestyle factors, a large one being stress. As vegan diets are often associated with religious practices, exercise (such as yoga) and meditation – some of which have been linked with improved mood – it may mean that vegans are improving their mental health through lifestyle rather than dietary means, but veganism is taking some of the credit. The best thing to do if you are struggling with your mental health is to seek professional advice from your doctor.

What people say: Veganism can help with arthritis

Myth or fact: It's complicated

There is some evidence that switching to a very low-fat vegan diet may improve certain symptoms for people who suffer from moderate-to-severe rheumatoid arthritis. As for osteoarthritis, the risk of getting this condition is significantly increased if you are overweight or obese. If switching to a vegan diet helps you to lose weight, then it is feasible that a vegan diet could improve joint pain in osteoarthritis, although this has not been proven.

What people say: Veganism improves fertility

Myth or fact: Myth

There is no evidence that a vegan diet can help with your fertility. However, there are also some lifestyle and dietary factors that we know can help, and these can be included within the vegan lifestyle. Firstly, it is important to make sure you are not suffering from excess stress and you are doing the recommended amount of exercise. Being overweight can also reduce fertility for both men and women, as does smoking, drinking alcohol excessively or taking illegal drugs. Eating a diet rich in carbohydrates, fruits, vegetables, fibre and antioxidants has been found to increase semen quality in men, and having plenty of antioxidants and not excessive amounts of fat or protein has been found to be helpful in women. Switching to a vegan diet is unlikely to be the magic answer, but there are definitely elements to a well-balanced diet that can be included in the vegan diet, which may help. If you are having issues with fertility, seeking medical advice is often really important.

How to eat vegan the right way

Although a well-balanced vegan diet can be healthy, sticking a vegan label on a diet does not automatically make it so – vodka, fizzy drinks and French fries are vegan but they're definitely not marketed as healthy foods. In the vegan diet there are five main food groups, and it is important that you are getting enough of each one, every day. These are fruits and vegetables, carbohydrate staples, protein-rich foods, fatty foods and calcium-rich (dairy alternative) foods.

FRUITS AND VEGETABLES

It is important to eat at least five portions of fruit or vegetables each day. A portion is 80g of fresh or 30g of dried fruits or vegetables. Fresh, tinned, frozen or dried all count towards your daily intake, and you should make sure you eat a wide variety of fruit and vegetables, as they all contain different vitamins and minerals. An easy way to do this is to make sure your plate is colourful at each meal. Eat the rainbow!

CARBOHYDRATES

Some people think carbohydrates will make you gain weight. This assumption is made for two reasons. Firstly, the rise in obesity in the UK and USA has been associated with a decrease in protein and fat consumption and an increase in eating carbohydrates. But it may in fact be the type of carbohydrate (e.g. sugary foods) that is the problem. Secondly, people who cut out carbs often do lose weight, because carbohydrates are found in many foods (including high-fat, high-sugar ones), and removing them from your diet often results in replacing them with fruits and vegetables.

But actually, carbohydrates are a crucial part of a balanced diet. Because a vegan diet involves cutting out foods that contain animal products, it is crucial not to restrict yourself any further. Each meal should be based upon a carbohydrate food such as:

- Rice
- Starchy vegetables (such as potatoes or sweet potatoes)
- Pasta
- Oats
- Bread
- Grains (such as quinoa, buckwheat or couscous)
- Breakfast cereals – some are very high in sugar, so check the label!

N.B. To make sure you get the recommended 30g per day of fibre, it is best to choose wholegrain varieties of these carbs, such as brown rice, brown pasta and brown bread.

PROTEIN-RICH FOODS

Often people who are choosing to try a vegan lifestyle are most worried about whether they will get enough protein. You may need to put a bit more effort into your diet to make sure you meet your protein needs than you would do if you followed an omnivorous diet, but it is definitely achievable. Every recipe in this book has been carefully designed to include a good source of vegan protein.

The right amount of protein for you will depend on your age, weight and exercise goals. Generally, an adult who lives a fairly sedentary lifestyle will need 0.75g per kilogram of body weight per day. For example, if you weigh 70kg you will need to eat 53g per day (70 x 0.75). This is best consumed across the course of the day, so your body can use it to the best of its ability. On a vegan diet, many sources of protein (such as meat, fish, dairy and eggs) are excluded, so it is important to make sure you are getting it from other sources. These include:

- Beans
- Lentils
- Chickpeas
- Nuts
- Seeds
- Soya products (such as milk, yoghurt, tofu and tempeh)

If you're an athlete with a busy training schedule, you can still meet your energy and protein requirements on a vegan diet. There are even many internationally renowned athletes who have followed a vegan diet, such as the amazing Venus and Serena Williams, who have both been ranked women's world no1 singles players during their careers. The exact amount of protein an athlete needs is under debate, and what might be enough for one athlete may not be enough for another. For example, it may be easier to meet the needs of a speed and agility athlete (e.g.

runner, hockey player, yoga-lover) than the needs of a strength athlete (e.g. weight lifter, rugby or American football player). Other factors for an athlete to consider are the micronutrients listed below – calcium, vitamin D, iron, B12 and iodine. One study found no demonstrative benefit for an athlete to consume more than 2g per kg per day of protein, and, in fact, excess protein may negatively affect calcium stores, kidney function, bone health and cardiovascular health.

Generally in the western world, we are at higher risk of having protein intakes that are too high rather than too low. For the majority of people who do moderate exercise, all the recipes in this book will give you enough protein.

SOURCES OF FAT

It is absolutely essential to include fat in the diet. Fat is not only an important source of calories, it is also essential for the healthy functioning of all the cells in our body – the outside of the cell (the membrane) contains fat and allows the cell to function properly.

There are three types of fat: saturated, polyunsaturated and monounsaturated. As a general rule of thumb, saturated fats are not good for our heart, while mono- and polyunsaturated fats are. This is because saturated fat increases your 'bad' cholesterol (fat in the blood), while unsaturated fats can reduce your 'bad' cholesterol and/or increase your 'good' cholesterol. Fat should provide no more than 35 per cent of our total energy intake per day, with a maximum of 10 per cent coming from saturated fats. If you find that you are accidentally losing weight on a vegan diet and don't want to be, focusing on getting enough healthy fats in the diet is a good way to combat this.

Most saturated fats are found in animal sources, so naturally the vegan diet is much lower in these than a vegetarian or omnivorous diet. Hence why a vegan diet could be good for your heart, as it may have a beneficial effect on your cholesterol! However, some plant sources of fat, such as coconut and palm oil, are also saturated, so are best enjoyed in moderation.

Sources of monounsaturated fats include:

- Most vegetable oils, such as sunflower, hazelnut, olive, canola, almond, peanut, corn, sesame and soya bean.
- Avocados and olives. Some nuts, such as hazelnuts, macadamias, pecans, almonds, pistachios and cashews. Therefore including nut butters (such as peanut, almond or cashew) or tahini (sesame paste) will be good for your heart.

In this book, avocados, nut butter, tahini and olive oil feature heavily, partly because they are delicious and partly because of their beneficial effect on the heart. You should make sure you include nuts and seeds in your diet every day to get enough heart-healthy fats.

Polyunsaturated fats are good for your heart, too. There are two main types – omega 3 and omega 6. Polyunsaturated fats not only have a beneficial effect on cholesterol, but long-chain omega 3 polyunsaturated fats also have an effect on the electrical impulses in your heart and therefore your heartbeat. Good sources of polyunsaturated fats include:

- Flaxseed oil (linseed oil is the same thing)
- Walnuts
- Canola and soya bean oils
- Soya products
- Hempseed-based beverages
- Spirulina

Pregnant or lactating women have particularly high needs for omega 3, so they would benefit from using long-chain omega 3 supplements. These are made from algae and can be found in all good health-food stores or on the internet. If you want to choose an appropriate supplement, make sure you consult a doctor, dietitian or Association for Nutrition registered nutritionist, as there are many supplements available that either are of no benefit, or could even have a negative impact on your health.

CALCIUM-RICH FOODS

As I explained on page 12, it is essential that we get enough calcium in the diet, as it is crucial for bone health. The vegan diet cuts out many high-calcium food sources (e.g. dairy products) so it is really important to find other alternatives. Good vegan sources include:

- Calcium-fortified plant milk (see below for different types)
- Tofu
- Tempeh
- Calcium-fortified cereal
- Tahini
- Calcium-fortified bread (wholemeal bread, pitta, chapattis, etc.)
- Broccoli and spring greens

'Fortified' just means that a nutrient has been added into the food (in this case, calcium has been added). Organic foods are not fortified, so from a health perspective it is better to buy non-organic dairy alternatives so you get more calcium. Of course, some people want to stick to organic dairy alternatives. If that is you, it might be worth considering taking a supplement. Make sure you include a good source of calcium every day in your diet (three portions of calcium-rich foods are required per day for children).

There are lots of different plant milks available; your choice will depend on taste and what nutrients are important for you in your diet. Provided you buy milks fortified with calcium, they are a great source of this essential mineral. But what else is there to consider?

Milk type	Details
Soya milk	Soya milk has a similar level of protein to cow's milk, so it is a good milk option for people with high protein requirements (e.g. athletes or children).
Almond, hemp, rice, coconut, hazelnut and oat	All popular choices, as many people like the taste. They are generally all low in calories, fat and protein, all of which are essential for a healthy diet, so you must make sure you get these essential nutrients from elsewhere. For example, if you are making a smoothie with almond milk, ensure there is another good source of protein in there. N.B. Coconut milk often contains rice milk (see below), so check the packet before giving to children.
Rice milk	Rice milk is not safe to give to children under 4½ years old due to the high arsenic content, which can be damaging. It is fine in adults, though, as the arsenic content is low enough for our kidneys to remove it.

EXTRA: VITAMINS AND MINERALS

Finally, when you are going vegan there will be certain vitamins and minerals in your diet that you will need to give extra thought to. This is because the vitamins and minerals listed below are found in high quantities in meat and dairy, so when following a vegan diet you must look for other sources. Here I've given the vitamins and minerals you should look out for, and which foods you can find them in. If you are looking for a vegan supplement in health-food stores, make sure it contains these vitamins and minerals.

Vitamin D

Everyone in the UK is at risk of vitamin D deficiency! Intakes of this essential vitamin can come from fortified foods (e.g. breakfast cereals*) and from sunshine, so people with reduced exposure to the outdoors and natural day light are at higher risk of a deficiency – such as the elderly, who may not go outside as often; people who cover their skin for religious reasons; people with dark skin; or people who use plenty of suncream. The UK recommends an intake of 10ug daily of vitamin D for everyone – and in this country to ensure you reach that amount you need a supplement. Low levels of vitamin D have been associated with increased risk of certain cancers, poor bone health and can impact mental health. Deficiency is often higher in the vegan population compared to non-vegans.

* A note on breakfast cereals – many are extremely sugary, so it is important that you read the label for sugar content.

Iron

As I explained on page 14, there are two types of iron – heme and non-heme. Vegans have low intakes of heme iron, and high intakes of non-heme iron, so need to have plenty of vitamin C in the diet to absorb the iron they eat. Good sources of iron in a vegan diet are fortified breakfast cereals, fortified bread, baked beans, butter beans, tofu, tempeh, figs, apricots, Brazil nuts, peanut butter, dates, almonds, sesame seeds, sunflower seeds, hazelnuts, broccoli and spinach. Combining these foods with foods that are high in vitamin C is important. For example, you could have a glass of orange juice with your fortified cereal for breakfast, or sunflower seeds in your salad with a dressing containing lemon juice.

Vitamin B12

Deficiency in this important vitamin can cause neurological symptoms. Deficiency is more common in vegans, because one of the main sources of B12 in the diet is meat, which is, of course, avoided in the vegan diet. Therefore, make sure you add in other sources, such as fortified soya and rice beverages, certain breakfast cereals and meat analogues, and fortified nutritional yeast. Alternatively (or in addition), you should take a daily vitamin B12 supplement to make sure you meet your daily requirements.

Iodine

Iodine is needed to make the thyroid hormones; these regulate many body processes including growth and regulating metabolism, and are vital for the development of a baby's brain during pregnancy and early life. Following a vegan diet puts you at increased risk of iodine deficiency as many good food sources are animal products (dairy, meat, eggs and fish). When you are deficient in this important mineral, symptoms can include extreme fatigue, goitre, irritability, depression, low body temperature and reduced mental capability, so it's important to make sure you're getting enough. Iodine is found in the soil, so it seems surprising that vegans are more likely to be deficient than omnivores. However, the iodine in the soil is taken up by the plants, then eaten by animals then eaten by humans, and at each step of the food chain the iodine accumulates (this is called bio-accumulation). By not eating animals, you are going to consume less iodine.

Good vegan sources of iodine include dried fruits such as prunes, some vegetables, potatoes, nuts and seaweed.

How to use this book

RECIPE COUNT

The book contains 30 breakfasts, 30 lunches and 30 dinners, all organised in individual days over the course of four-and-a-half weeks. If you would rather choose recipes by breakfast, lunch and dinner, you can use the Recipe Index on page 238.

SHOPPING LIST

At the beginning of each week there is a shopping list which gives all the easy-to-source ingredients that you will need to make the recipes for the next seven days. The aim is to use up all the food you buy at the beginning of the week, with minimal waste – which is good for the planet and your pocket! Each week starts on the Saturday, to allow you to go to the shops at the beginning of the weekend (or on Friday night) so you are ready for the week ahead.

STORE CUPBOARD ESSENTIALS

The 'store cupboard essentials' section lists all the ingredients that are helpful to have in your cupboards at all times, and which you will use for many recipes throughout the book. In the first week you will need to invest in this list as well as the shopping list – but don't be put off! Anything you buy this week will save you time and hopefully money in the long run. And you might find you have lots of these ingredients in your cupboards already.

BATCH COOKING

To make this book as practical as possible, many of the lunches use ingredients that are leftover from dinner from the few days preceding, or are deliberately made in bulk to be split over a few days. For instance, where you make a walnut and kale pesto for dinner on Monday in Week 1 (page 56) it can be used as a delicious salad dressing for lunch on Tuesday (page 59).

SERVING SIZE

Each of the main meals (breakfast, lunch and dinner) are designed to serve two people, unless stated otherwise. Where they do serve more, indicated with this symbol 🥘, you can freeze the excess for another day. Freezing leftovers or cooking in bulk is another great way to make healthy eating easier and it can often be cheaper, too.

CALORIE COUNTS

I personally don't condone calorie counting, but I understand that it can be a useful tool for those who are trying to cut back or for those who need to make sure they're eating plenty. All of the recipes in this book have approximate calorie counts for one portion, but bear in mind that calories vary greatly depending on the size of the ingredients you're using and the brand of the product, so these are loose estimations.

SNACKS

As well as main meals, this book will also give you 10 snack ideas. These are not included within the weekly shopping list, as you may want to have them at any time throughout the month! If you find that your body needs more calories than the recipes in this book give you, snacks are a good way to fuel you and are often particularly important if you are exercising.

EQUIPMENT

To make this book as practical as possible, you should not need to invest in any fancy kitchen equipment. Below is a suggested list of essential items:
· Vegetable peeler
· Set of saucepans
· Ovenproof dish
· Baking tray
· Mixing bowl
· Wooden spoon
· Blender/smoothie maker: this is essential for smoothies, soups, sauces (e.g. katsu curry sauce, page 131) and energy bites
· Tupperware boxes and drink containers (if you want to take lunch or drinks into work)
  And nice to have but not essential:
· Spiraliser: if you don't have one, there's no need to buy one! Just use a peeler.

Store cupboard essentials

Oils, vinegars and sauces

- [ ] Olive oil
- [ ] Coconut oil
- [ ] Soy sauce
- [ ] White wine vinegar
- [ ] Tomato ketchup
- [ ] Balsamic vinegar
- [ ] Rice vinegar
- [ ] Yellow miso paste
- [ ] Horseradish sauce
- [ ] Pomegranate molasses
- [ ] Truffle-infused olive oil (optional – but not as expensive as you would expect and you can buy it easily from most supermarkets)

Fruit and nuts

- [ ] Capers
- [ ] Dried apricots
- [ ] Medjool dates
- [ ] Sesame seeds
- [ ] Linseeds
- [ ] Chia seeds
- [ ] Pistachio nuts
- [ ] Walnuts
- [ ] Pecans
- [ ] Peanuts
- [ ] Hazelnuts
- [ ] Flaked almonds

Carbohydrate staples

- [ ] Plain flour
- [ ] Rolled oats
- [ ] Quinoa
- [ ] Couscous
- [ ] Barley
- [ ] Buckwheat
- [ ] Dried wholewheat linguine/ spaghetti
- [ ] Dried penne (or other short pasta)
- [ ] Polenta/cornmeal
- [ ] Rice of your choice
- [ ] Risotto rice
- [ ] Wild rice
- [ ] Dried rice noodles

Herbs, flavourings and spices

- [ ] Agave nectar
- [ ] Maple syrup
- [ ] Balsamic glaze
- [ ] Tahini
- [ ] Thai red curry paste (buy the best one you can find, as this will have a huge impact on the flavour of the dishes you use it in)
- [ ] Harissa paste
- [ ] Tabasco sauce
- [ ] Sriracha sauce
- [ ] Za'atar
- [ ] Medium curry powder
- [ ] Cardamom pods
- [ ] Turmeric
- [ ] Mustard seeds
- [ ] Mixed spice
- [ ] Salt
- [ ] Pepper and black peppercorns
- [ ] Paprika
- [ ] Chilli flakes
- [ ] Cumin – ground

- [ ] Garlic (at least 5 bulbs)
- [ ] Dried oregano
- [ ] Dried rosemary
- [ ] Dried bay leaves
- [ ] Cinnamon – ground and sticks
- [ ] Coriander – ground and seeds
- [ ] Ground allspice
- [ ] Cardamom pods
- [ ] Moroccan spice mix
- [ ] Tomato purée
- [ ] Nutmeg – whole
- [ ] Raw cacao powder
- [ ] Vanilla extract

Other

- [ ] Vegetable stock cubes
- [ ] Nutritional yeast flakes
- [ ] Peanut butter (if you can, buy a good brand without added sugar)
- [ ] Dark muscovado sugar
- [ ] Soya protein powder (or other vegan alternative, if preferred)

- [ ] Baking powder
- [ ] Bran flakes
- [ ] Dry sherry (optional)
- [ ] Vegan yeast extract, e.g. Marmite/Vegemite
- [ ] Strong English breakfast tea bags

For the freezer

- [ ] Sliced sourdough bread (or other bread if you prefer!)
- [ ] Wholemeal pitta breads
- [ ] Peas
- [ ] Broad beans
- [ ] Root ginger (buy fresh, chop into knobs and freeze)

For the fridge

- [ ] Olive oil spread/vegan butter (make sure you check the nutrition information, as many margarines contain buttermilk)

Extra

- [ ] Tin foil
- [ ] Cling film
- [ ] Wooden skewers
- [ ] Tupperware boxes (if you want to take lunch to work)

Recipes: Week 1

N.B. Each meal serves two people
unless otherwise stated.

SHOPPING LIST

Dairy alternatives

- [ ] 1 litre coconut milk
- [ ] 250g pot of coconut yoghurt
- [ ] 1 litre hazelnut milk
- [ ] 1 litre soya milk

Fruit and vegetables

- [ ] 3 white onions
- [ ] 4 red onions
- [ ] 6 sweet potatoes
- [ ] 550g cherry tomatoes
- [ ] 5 plum tomatoes
- [ ] 5 avocados
- [ ] 2 courgettes
- [ ] 1 pak choi*
- [ ] 100g tenderstem broccoli*
- [ ] 100g baby corn*
- [ ] 100g sugar snap peas*
- [ ] 3 red peppers
- [ ] 200g asparagus
- [ ] 120g bag of rocket
- [ ] 150g kale
- [ ] 1 celery head (keep 3 sticks for week 2)
- [ ] 1 butternut squash
- [ ] 1 leek
- [ ] 1 carrot
- [ ] 620g chestnut mushrooms
- [ ] Small box pomegranate seeds
- [ ] 1 chilli pepper
- [ ] 4 small-medium bananas
- [ ] 500g bag of frozen mango chunks
- [ ] 500g blackberries (fresh or frozen)
- [ ] 200g fresh raspberries
- [ ] 3 limes
- [ ] 3 lemons

Carbohydrate staples

- [ ] 2 bread rolls
- [ ] 8 flour tortilla wraps (freeze the 4 left over separately, laid flat in large sandwich bags)

Dried fruit, nuts and seeds

- ☐ 200g desiccated coconut
- ☐ 250g dried fruit and nut mix **
- ☐ 350g dried mixed fruit

Other

- ☐ 1 x 435g tin refried beans
- ☐ 2 x 400g tins chickpeas
- ☐ 100g silken tofu
- ☐ 1 x 400g tin pinto beans
- ☐ 1 x 400g tin chopped tomatoes
- ☐ 250g ready cooked puy lentils
- ☐ 1 x 400g tin black beans
- ☐ 1 x 198g tin sweetcorn
- ☐ 500g firm tofu
- ☐ White wine of your choice (at least 70ml)

Fresh herbs

- ☐ Coriander***
- ☐ Parsley***
- ☐ Mint***
- ☐ Thyme***
- ☐ Rosemary***
- ☐ Lemongrass stalk

*Often you can buy these ingredients together in a stir-fry pack, which is cheaper and reduces waste

**If you want to make your own fruit and nut mix, you need to buy the following:

- ☐ 20g sesame seeds
- ☐ 50g sunflower seeds
- ☐ 20g linseeds
- ☐ 50g hazelnuts
- ☐ 50g dried sour cherries
- ☐ 20g chia seeds
- ☐ 40g sultanas

***I would suggest buying a pot of these herbs rather than a packet – they will keep for longer and be cheaper in the long run.

MENU

	Breakfast	Lunch	Dinner
Saturday	Mexican brunch bowl	Butternut squash bisque	Savoury oatmeal with sautéed mushrooms and thyme
Sunday	Currant tea loaf with homemade jam	Spiced carrot, date and lentil salad	Chilli non-carne with hummus and avocado
Monday	Mango and coconut smoothie	Sweet potato 'Tex-Mex' salad	Roast vegetable and polenta tart with kale and walnut pesto
Tuesday	Sourdough toast with peanut butter and homemade chia jam	Roasted vegetable and pesto pasta salad	Aromatic crispy tofu stir-fry

	Breakfast	Lunch	Dinner
Wednesday	Toasted muesli with dried fruit and nuts	Crispy tofu, hummus and avocado pitta	Sweet potato falafel with jewelled couscous
Thursday	Mango and coconut chia pudding	Falafel wrap	Quinoa bowl – baked asparagus, cherry tomatoes, peppers with hummus and balsamic glaze
Friday	Banana, maple syrup and pecan porridge	Mediterran-ean-inspired sandwiches	Linguine with a mushroom and chestnut sauce

BREAKFAST

Mexican brunch bowl

Under 600 calories

This brunch bowl is wonderfully colourful and very easy to make. Don't be put off by the long list of ingredients – you assemble each part separately and then pile everything together into the tortilla. This recipe also works as fajitas in the evening.

FOR THE SALSA
3 ripe plum tomatoes, roughly
    chopped
1 medium white onion, roughly
    chopped
2 garlic cloves, roughly
    chopped
½ tbsp olive oil
Pinch of chilli flakes
Small bunch of coriander
Salt and pepper, to taste

FOR THE HERBY TOMATOES
250g cherry tomatoes

1 tbsp olive oil
2 garlic cloves, crushed
1 tbsp dried oregano

FOR THE GUACAMOLE
1 avocado, halved and stoned
Juice of 1 lime
½ tbsp olive oil
Tabasco sauce, to taste

TO SERVE
1 x 435g tin refried beans
2 flour tortilla wraps
1 lime, cut into wedges

1. Preheat the oven to 200°C/180°C fan/400°F/gas mark 6.

2. Start by making the salsa. Combine the chopped tomatoes, onion and garlic with the olive oil, chilli flakes, salt and pepper in a small saucepan and cook for 15–20 minutes until the onion starts to brown. Take off the heat and allow to cool, then blitz with most of the coriander, saving a few leaves to garnish, using a hand-held blender in the pan, or transfer to a blender and blitz until slightly chunky.

3. Next make the herby cherry tomatoes. Tip the tomatoes into a baking tin with the olive oil, garlic and oregano and season with salt and pepper, then roast in the oven for 15–20 minutes until soft.

4. To make the guacamole, scoop out the avocado and mash it in a bowl with the lime juice, olive oil, some salt and pepper and Tabasco to taste.

5. When you are ready to serve, heat the refried beans in a small saucepan over a medium heat according to the instructions on the tin.

6. Heat the tortillas according to the packet instructions, then lay them in two large pasta bowls or on plates. Pile each one high with warm refried beans, guacamole, the herby tomatoes and salsa. Serve with the lime wedges, scattered with the reserved coriander leaves.

LUNCH

Butternut squash bisque

Under 500 calories

This soup is a delicious winter warmer and a real crowd pleaser.
The butternut squash takes 90 minutes to cook, so put this
in the oven well in advance and do something else while it
is cooking. The sherry is optional, but it makes it taste extra
special! This will make a larger quantity than you need, but it
freezes well so put the excess into airtight containers and
store ready for future lunches!

1 medium-sized butternut squash	125ml dry sherry (optional)
1 tbsp olive oil	½ tsp grated nutmeg
1 medium white onion, diced	2 vegetable stock cubes, dissolved in 1 litre boiling water
1 leek, diced	
½ tsp ground cumin	Salt and pepper, to taste
2 garlic cloves, diced	
1 thumb-sized piece of root ginger, grated	TO SERVE
2 tbsp maple syrup	Handful of coriander leaves, chopped
2 tbsp soy sauce	2 bread rolls, warmed

1. Preheat the oven to 190°C/170°C fan/375°F/gas mark 5.

2. Prick the skin of the butternut squash all over, then place the whole vegetable in a roasting tin lined with tin foil and cook in the oven for 90 minutes, until very soft.

3. Allow the butternut squash to cool then cut in half and remove the seeds and stringy insides. Scoop out the flesh, discarding any stray seeds, stringy insides and skin.

4. In a large saucepan, heat the olive oil and brown the onion. Add the leek and cumin and cook for a few minutes until softened and slightly browned, then add the garlic and ginger and cook for another few minutes. Pour in the maple syrup, soy sauce, sherry (if using) and nutmeg. Finally, add the squash and the stock.

5. Bring the stock to the boil and simmer for 15 minutes, so that all the ingredients are lovely and soft and the liquid is well infused with all the flavours.

6. Use a hand-held blender or transfer to a blender and purée until smooth. If the soup is a little thick, add more boiling water until you reach the desired consistency.

7. Serve scattered with coriander with some warmed bread rolls alongside.

DINNER

Savoury oatmeal with sautéed mushrooms and thyme

Under 600 calories

Porridge is often thought of as a sweet breakfast food, served with fruit and syrups, but traditionally it was made simply with water and salt. There's no reason why oats can't be enjoyed throughout the day, and they are a great source of soluble fibre.

120g rolled oats
480ml soya milk
1 tsp salt
1 tbsp olive oil
1 medium white onion, diced
2 garlic cloves, minced
220g chestnut mushrooms, sliced

3 sprigs of thyme, leaves removed and chopped
3 sprigs of rosemary, leaves removed and chopped
2 tsp nutritional yeast flakes
Pepper, to taste
2 tbsp truffle-infused olive oil, to serve

1. In a pan over a low heat, combine the oats, milk and salt and cook for 15–20 minutes, so that the oats absorb all the moisture. Do this nice and slowly so that the oats become creamier.

2. In a saucepan over a medium heat, heat the olive oil then add the onion and garlic. Sauté for about 3 minutes until they begin to soften. Add the mushrooms, thyme and rosemary and cook until the mushrooms are golden brown and slightly crispy on the outside.

3. When the oatmeal is cooked through, stir in the nutritional yeast flakes.

4. Serve the crispy mushrooms in bowls topped with the creamy oatmeal, lots of pepper and a drizzle of truffle-infused olive oil.

Get ahead!

Tonight, you will need to prepare the jam and part of the tea loaf for breakfast tomorrow so make sure you take a look at Sunday's recipes.

BREAKFAST

Currant tea loaf with homemade jam

Makes roughly 8 slices – each slice with jam under 400 calories

This recipe feels like a real treat – and any leftovers are great for snacks. The homemade jam uses chia seeds rather than sugar to bind the fruit together, which means it is lower in sugar but it doesn't keep for as long as normal jam (sugar preserves the fruit), so it should be used within a week. You do need to make the jam one day ahead, to allow the chia seeds to absorb the moisture and swell.

Store the jam in a sterilised jar in the fridge. To sterilise a jar, wash it and its lid in hot soapy water then stand both upside down in a roasting tin while they're still wet. Put the tin in an oven preheated to 170°C/150°C fan/325°F/gas mark 3 for about 15 minutes. Use the jar immediately.

FOR THE TEA LOAF

2 bags of strong English
    breakfast tea
350g dried mixed fruit
150g dark muscovado sugar
300ml boiling water
250g plain flour
¼ tsp salt
1 tsp mixed spice
2 tsp baking powder
75g vegan butter, plus extra
    to serve
100ml hazelnut milk

FOR THE JAM

500g blackberries (fresh
    or frozen)
½ tsp vanilla extract
30g chia seeds

EQUIPMENT

1 x 450g loaf tin – lined with
    baking parchment or greased
    with vegan butter

---

1. The night before you make the loaf, put the tea bags in a heatproof bowl large enough to hold all the ingredients, and add the dried mixed fruit and sugar. Pour over the boiling water and cover loosely with a clean, dry tea towel.

2. Also the night before, make the jam. In a small saucepan, gently heat the blackberries for 5 minutes. When soft, mash them with a fork or potato masher.

3. Add the vanilla extract and chia seeds, stir over the heat for a further few minutes. Remove the saucepan from the heat and tip the jam into a sterilised jar, seal and once cool, store in the fridge.

4. The following day, preheat the oven to 170°C/150°C fan/325°F/gas mark 3.

5. Remove the teabags from the fruit mixture and discard. The fruit should have absorbed most of the liquid now, so there's no need to drain it.

6. Sift the flour, salt, mixed spice and baking powder into the bowl with the sugary fruit mixture.

7. Melt the vegan butter in a small saucepan, then add this to the batter mix in the bowl. Pour in the hazelnut milk and mix thoroughly.

8. Transfer the batter to the prepared tin and bake for 1 hour– 1 hour 15 minutes until well risen and dark golden brown. If you insert a cocktail stick into the centre of the loaf, it should come out clean.

9. Leave the tea loaf to cool in the tin for 15 minutes, before transferring it to a wire rack. You can either leave it to cool completely before eating it, or slice it warm and serve with vegan butter and homemade chia jam.

LUNCH

Spiced carrot, date and lentil salad

Under 500 calories

This salad is very quick to make – I've chosen a light lunch for today as you may be quite full from the tea loaf at breakfast! The flavour combinations are unusual but lovely, and you don't even need to cook it, so it really couldn't be easier.

---

1 tbsp olive oil
½ tsp ground cumin
½ tsp mustard seeds
1 garlic clove, minced
250g ready cooked puy lentils
1 carrot, coarsely grated

100g sesame seeds
Small bunch of coriander,
   roughly chopped
100g medjool dates, pitted and
   chopped

---

1. In a pan over a medium heat, heat the olive oil and add the cumin, mustard seeds and garlic. Cook for a few minutes until the garlic is soft.

2. Mix all the other ingredients together thoroughly in a large serving bowl, then pour over the hot, fragrant garlic oil just before serving.

DINNER

Chilli non-carne with hummus and avocado

Under 600 calories

This is an incredibly easy recipe to make, with very little washing-up. As the chilli contains sweet potato, I find that I don't need rice as well, as it's pretty filling, but if you are really hungry, do serve it with some. You'll be using the hummus for other recipes in the week, so make sure you only use a tablespoon for each bowl.

FOR THE CHILLI
1 tbsp olive oil
2 garlic cloves, minced
1 red onion, diced
2 celery sticks, diced
1 sweet potato, diced
200g chestnut mushrooms, sliced
1 red pepper, deseeded and diced
2 tbsp tomato purée
2 tsp dried oregano
1 tsp paprika
1 tsp chilli flakes
1 tsp yeast extract, e.g. Marmite/Vegemite
1 x 400g tin pinto beans, drained and rinsed

1 x 400g tin chopped tomatoes
Salt and pepper, to taste

FOR THE HUMMUS
1 x 400g tin chickpeas, drained and rinsed
3 tbsp olive oil
Juice of 1 lemon
2 tsp tahini
1 tsp paprika
1 tsp ground cumin

TO SERVE
1 avocado, halved, stoned, peeled and sliced
Small bunch of coriander, finely chopped

1. Over a medium heat, heat the olive oil in a large saucepan, then add the garlic, onion, celery and sweet potato. Cook until softened, about 5 minutes.

2. Add the mushrooms and pepper and cook for a further 5 minutes.

3. Add the tomato purée, oregano, paprika, chilli flakes and Marmite. Stir until all the vegetables are well coated in the purée and spices.

4. Pour in the beans and chopped tomatoes. Fill the tomato tin half full with water and pour this into the pan.

5. Simmer, with the lid on, for about 45 minutes so that all the flavours develop, checking regularly to make sure none of the chilli is catching on the bottom. If necessary, add more liquid.

6. After 45 minutes the sauce should be thick and the chilli very aromatic. If it looks a little watery, cook it a bit longer with the lid off. Add salt and pepper to taste.

7. Meanwhile, make the hummus. Tip the chickpeas, olive oil, lemon juice, tahini, paprika and cumin into a blender and blitz together until completely smooth. Add about 3 tablespoons of water, a small amount at a time, until you reach the desired consistency.

8. Serve the chilli with sliced avocado, a tablespoon of hummus each (save the rest for later recipes, ideally in a sterilised jar) and a sprinkling of chopped coriander.

Get ahead!

If you have the time, cook the sweet potato tonight for tomorrow's lunch – Sweet potato 'Tex-Mex' salad.

You can also steep the soya milk with the herbs and spices overnight if you want a stronger herby flavour.

BREAKFAST

Mango and coconut smoothie

Under 550 calories

Smoothies are good things to have in the morning, provided they contain a good source of protein, carbohydrate and also a calcium alternative (see food groups, page 17).

400ml coconut milk
125g (½ pot) coconut yoghurt
2 small bananas
250g frozen mango chunks

2 scoops soya protein powder
(or other vegan alternative,
if preferred)

---

1. Combine all the ingredients in a blender and blitz until smooth and thoroughly mixed.

2. Divide into two glasses and serve.

LUNCH

Sweet potato 'Tex-Mex' salad

Under 550 calories

This is a great quick lunch for taking in to work, but the sweet potato needs to either be cooked the night before or first thing in the morning.

1 sweet potato, peeled and cut into even chunks

1 tbsp olive oil

1 tsp chilli flakes

1 x 400g tin black beans, drained and rinsed

1 x 198g tin sweetcorn, drained

1 avocado, halved, stoned, peeled and cut into chunks

2 plum tomatoes, cut into chunks

1 red onion, thinly sliced

Juice of 1 lime

Small bunch of coriander, finely chopped

1. Preheat the oven to 180°C/160°C fan/350°F/gas mark 4.

2. On a baking tray, toss the sweet potato chunks in the olive oil and scatter over the chilli flakes, then roast for 25 minutes, or until tender.

3. Either let the sweet potato cool before mixing with all the other ingredients in a large serving bowl, or toss everything together while it is still warm and and serve immediately.

DINNER

Roast vegetable and polenta tart with kale and walnut pesto

Under 500 calories

This tart is a real showstopper! Steeping the soya milk with the herbs and spices is really important; the further in advance you can do this, the better, because leaving the soya milk to steep will give a stronger herby flavour.

If you don't want to make your own pesto, you can buy it fresh from many supermarkets. Have a look in the fresh pasta section of the supermarket and read the ingredients to make sure it's vegan – many shop-bought pestos contain parmesan.

FOR THE POLENTA
400ml soya milk
1 tsp black peppercorns
2 sprigs of rosemary
1 bay leaf
100g polenta

FOR THE ROASTED
VEGETABLES
2 courgettes, cut into half-
    moon chunks
2 red onions, cut into half
    moons

4 garlic cloves, crushed
2 sweet potatoes, peeled and
    cut into cubes
1 tbsp olive oil
Salt and pepper, to taste

FOR THE PESTO
150g kale, large stems removed
50g walnuts, toasted
2 garlic cloves, peeled
Juice and zest of 1 lemon
150ml olive oil

---

1. Preheat the oven to 180°C/160°C fan/350°F/gas mark 4.

2. On the hob, heat the soya milk with the peppercorns, rosemary sprigs and bay leaf until almost boiling, then take off the heat and allow to cool and let the flavours infuse.

3. Meanwhile, combine the vegetables, garlic, olive oil and salt and pepper in a 20cm square ovenproof baking dish. Bake in the oven for 30 minutes.

4. When the vegetables have baked for 25 minutes, strain the soya milk to remove the herbs and peppercorns and pour into a saucepan. Then add the polenta, a small amount at a time, to the herby soya milk and whisk over a medium heat, until all the moisture is absorbed and the polenta is cooked through. You may need some extra liquid, depending on the instructions on the packet, as all polenta differs. You can add more boiling water from the kettle if you need to.

5. To make the pesto, blitz together all the dry ingredients in a blender. Add the lemon zest and juice and then the olive oil, a little at a time, while the blender is running, until well combined.

6. When the roasted vegetables are done, keep half back for lunch on Tuesday (store in a clean Tupperware or other sealable pot in the fridge). Pour the polenta over the rest of the vegetables and return to the oven for 20 minutes.

7. Serve hot, drizzled with pesto. You'll have much more pesto than you need, so put the rest in a sterilised jar (see page 46), add a thin (approx. ¼cm) layer of olive oil on top to seal, and keep in the fridge.

BREAKFAST

Sourdough toast with peanut butter and homemade chia jam

Under 500 calories

As you've made the jam already (see page 46), this couldn't be easier. It also makes a great snack and it's good for lunch.

4 slices of sourdough bread	2 tbsp homemade chia jam
4 tbsp peanut butter	(see page 46)

1. Toast the sourdough.

2. Spread each slice with peanut butter, followed by homemade chia jam.

LUNCH

Roasted vegetable and pesto pasta salad

Under 500 calories

This lunch uses the pesto and roasted vegetables that you made for dinner on Monday, so it takes very little preparation. I've suggested using dried pasta throughout the book, as fresh pasta often contains egg. However, if you do find vegan fresh pasta and you'd rather use that, it will be delicious, too.

150g pasta
Roasted vegetables (leftover
   from dinner on Monday)
½ bag of ready-washed rocket

4 tbsp pesto (leftover from
   dinner on Monday)
Salt and pepper, to taste

---

1. Cook the pasta according to the packet instructions. Drain.

2. Combine the roasted vegetables, drained pasta and rocket together.

3. Drizzle the pesto over the top and season with salt and pepper to taste.

DINNER

Aromatic crispy tofu stir-fry

Under 550 calories

Stir-frys are the real 'cheat' of the dinner world – they are incredibly easy to make, contain lots of healthy veggies and cooking this way requires very little washing-up. You can always vary the choice of vegetables. Here the veg are partially pan-fried and partially steamed, which is a traditional Chinese method of cooking.

Half the tofu should be kept back and stored in the fridge for Thursday's lunch.

200g dried rice noodles
500g firm tofu
2 tbsp olive oil
1 tbsp sesame seeds
1 chilli pepper, diced
1 lemongrass stalk, diced
1 garlic clove, minced
1 pak choi, sliced into ribbons

100g Tenderstem broccoli, cut in half lengthways
100g baby corn, cut in half lengthways
100g sugar snap peas, ends trimmed
2 tbsp peanut butter
100ml water

1. Preheat the oven to 200°C/180°C fan/400°F/gas mark 6.

2. Cook the rice noodles according to the packet instructions and set aside.

3. Cut the tofu into chunks and pat them dry with kitchen towel, then place on a baking tray lined with non-stick baking parchment, brush with 1 tablespoon of olive oil and sprinkle with the sesame seeds. Bake until golden, about 25 minutes, then remove from the oven. (Put half in a clean Tupperware or sealable pot and keep in the fridge for Thursday's lunch.)

4. Place the remaining olive oil in a wok over a medium heat. Add the chilli, lemongrass and garlic, and stir-fry for a few minutes until aromatic, ensuring the garlic doesn't catch and start to burn.

5. Add the remaining vegetables and cook for another 5 minutes, until the vegetables are soft. Add the peanut butter and water and mix to make a sauce, before adding the rice noodles and half the tofu to the pan.

6. Heat through thoroughly before serving.

BREAKFAST

Toasted muesli with dried fruit and nuts

This makes approx. 10 servings of muesli and contains under 250 calories per muesli serving and under 600 calories per serving with the accompaniments.

Toasting the bran flakes gives this straightforward breakfast a wonderful aroma and a delicious nutty flavour. It is really important to have slow-release carbohydrates at breakfast, and bran flakes are a really great source. This muesli will keep in an airtight container for a few weeks.

250g bran flakes
250g dried fruit and nut mix*

TO SERVE
125g coconut yoghurt
200g raspberries
100ml coconut milk
50g desiccated coconut,
   to decorate

* If you are feeling particularly adventurous, you can make your own fruit and nut mix!
I would recommend the following:
20g sesame seeds
50g sunflower seeds
20g linseeds
40g sultanas
50g hazelnuts
50g dried sour cherries
20g chia seeds

---

1. Preheat the oven to 180°C/160°C fan/350°F/gas mark 4.

2. Place the bran flakes in a shallow frying pan over a low heat and gently toast them, shaking the pan occasionally – you will be able to smell a lovely aroma as they are cooking, but be careful they don't burn. This will only take a few minutes. Tip out into a bowl.

3. Combine the dried fruit and nut mix with the bran flakes. Once cool, transfer to an airtight container.

4. Serve 50g of the muesli per person with the coconut yoghurt, fresh raspberries and coconut milk, and scatter with the dessicated coconut.

LUNCH

Crispy tofu, hummus and avocado pitta

Under 650 calories

I really enjoy this lunch when the pittas are warm and toasted. However, if you want to take this to work with you where you won't have a toaster available, that's OK, too – either have them untoasted, or you can toast them before you leave the house and have them crispy but not hot.

2 pitta breads
4 tbsp hummus (leftover from Sunday's dinner)

Crispy tofu (leftover from Tuesday's dinner)
1 avocado, halved, stoned, peeled and sliced

1. Toast the pittas.

2. Divide the remaining ingredients among the toasted pittas.

DINNER

Sweet potato falafel with jewelled couscous

Under 650 calories

Falafel is made from chickpeas, so makes a great source of protein for vegan diets. If you don't have the time or inclination to make falafel, it is very easy to buy from most supermarkets.

FOR THE FALAFEL

2 sweet potatoes, peeled and
   cubed

2 tbsp olive oil

1 tsp chilli flakes (optional)

1 x 400g tin chickpeas, drained
   and rinsed

1 tbsp za'atar

Handful of parsley, chopped

Handful of mint, chopped

FOR THE COUSCOUS

70g couscous

50g dried apricots, chopped

Handful of parsley, chopped

2 tbsp pomegranate seeds

50g pistachio nuts, shelled

1. Preheat the oven to 200°C/180°C fan/400°F/gas mark 6.

2. Spread out the sweet potatoes on a baking tray, drizzle with the olive oil and scatter over the chilli flakes, if using, then bake for 20 minutes, until really soft.

3. Put the sweet potatoes into the blender with the chickpeas, za'atar and chopped herbs. Blitz until smooth, then remove from the blender and shape into 12 small balls with your hands.

4. Put the raw falafel balls back onto the baking tray and return to the oven for another 15 minutes.

5. Prepare the couscous according to the packet instructions. Toss all the remaining ingredients through the couscous.

6. Set aside half of the falafel for lunch tomorrow (pop it in the fridge in a clean Tupperware or sealable pot). Serve the remaining falafel on a bed of the couscous.

Get ahead!

You need to start preparing tomorrow's breakfast tonight by soaking the chia seeds. You could do this while the falafel is baking.

BREAKFAST

Mango and coconut chia pudding

Under 600 calories

This breakfast reminds me of being on holiday – it's a great way to start the day. It takes a little preparation the night before – including leaving the chia seeds to swell overnight and defrosting the mango pieces – but it's worth it as that will save you time in the morning. Chia seeds are a very good source of soluble fibre, which is essential for keeping your bowels regular, and it also has beneficial effects on cholesterol.

500ml coconut milk
60g chia seeds
2 tbsp agave nectar
½ tsp vanilla extract

250g mango chunks, defrosted
Pinch of desiccated coconut,
   to decorate

---

1. Mix together the coconut milk, chia seeds, agave and vanilla extract in a jar or bowl. Refrigerate for 15 minutes then mix again. Cover the bowl or jar with a lid or cling film and return to the fridge overnight.

2. In the morning, remove the chia pudding from the fridge, layer half of it with half the chopped defrosted mango in a glass jar, then repeat until you have two layers of both the chia pudding and the mango.

3. Scatter with desiccated coconut to serve.

LUNCH

Falafel wrap

Under 700 calories

Falafel wraps are popular street food – and much healthier than their meaty cousins, the kebab. This makes a great lunch and if you're using leftovers from previous days it is very easy to put together.

---

2 flour tortilla wraps
6 falafels (leftover from
    Wednesday's dinner)
4 tbsp hummus (leftover from
    Saturday's dinner)

½ bag of ready-washed rocket
1 avocado, halved, stoned,
    peeled and sliced

---

1. Heat the tortillas according to the packet instructions, then lay them out on two plates and pile with the falafel, hummus, rocket and avocado.

2. Fold and roll the wraps ready to serve.

DINNER

Quinoa bowl – baked asparagus, cherry tomatoes, peppers with hummus and balsamic glaze

Under 500 calories

Quinoa bowls are, in my opinion, the ultimate comfort food but with a healthy twist. Quinoa is one of the few examples of a 'complete' vegan protein – that means it contains all the essential amino acids (the building blocks of protein). Adding hummus makes the bowl really creamy, while the vegetables still give it some 'crunch'.

2 red peppers, cut in half and deseeded
300g cherry tomatoes
200g asparagus
2 tbsp olive oil
2 tsp balsamic glaze

2 garlic cloves, crushed
Salt and pepper, to taste
120g quinoa
2 tbsp hummus (leftover from Saturday's dinner)

1. Preheat the oven to 200°C/180°C fan/400°F/gas mark 6.

2. Spread the peppers, cherry tomatoes and asparagus on a baking tray. Drizzle olive oil over all the vegetables and half the balsamic glaze over the asparagus. Crush the garlic into the peppers. Crack over the salt and pepper and bake in the oven for 25 minutes, until soft.

3. Cook the quinoa according to the packet instructions.

4. When the vegetables have finished cooking, set aside half of the peppers, asparagus and tomatoes for Friday's lunch.

5. Combine the remaining vegetables and the quinoa in a deep bowl and serve with 1 tablespoon of hummus per bowl and a drizzle of the remaining balsamic glaze.

BREAKFAST

Banana, maple syrup and pecan porridge

Under 600 calories each

This porridge involves putting everything in a pan and leaving it to simmer slowly. I often put this on the hob while getting ready to leave for work in the morning – just make sure you're never too far from an open flame...

80g rolled oats	½ tsp mixed spice
480ml hazelnut milk	2 tbsp maple syrup
2 medium bananas, chopped	50g pecans, roughly chopped

1. Put the oats, hazelnut milk, bananas and mixed spice into a saucepan over a low heat and cook for 5–10 minutes, until all the liquid is absorbed and the bananas are very soft. Stir regularly to stop the porridge sticking to the bottom of the saucepan.

2. Divide among two bowls, drizzle with the maple syrup and scatter over the chopped pecans.

LUNCH

Mediterranean-inspired sandwiches

Under 400 calories

I love the flavours in this sandwich – Mediterranean food is not only delicious, but the Mediterranean diet also has good evidence for heart health and reducing the risk of dementia. If you want to take your sandwiches to work and there isn't a toaster, you can have the pittas cold.

---

2 pitta breads
4 tbsp hummus (leftover from
    Saturday's dinner)

Peppers, tomatoes and
    asparagus (leftover from
    Thursday's dinner)

---

1. Toast the pitta breads and cut to open the breads.

2. Divide the ingredients between the pittas.

DINNER

Linguine with a mushroom and chestnut sauce

Under 500 calories

This pasta sauce is deliciously creamy – no one will believe you that it is vegan. This is a really good dish if you are trying out veganism for the first time, and are worried that you might miss creamy pasta sauces.

1 garlic clove, chopped

1 tsp olive oil

200g chestnut mushrooms, sliced

70ml white wine (the rest of the bottle can be drunk while cooking/eating!)

Juice of 1 lemon

100g silken tofu

3 tsp dried rosemary

Salt and pepper, to taste

A little water or soya milk (optional)

150g linguine (or other pasta shape)

60g walnuts, roughly chopped, to serve

1. Place a saucepan over a low heat and gently sauté the garlic in the olive oil until it is nicely aromatic but not browned.

2. Add the chestnut mushrooms and sauté until soft.

3. Add the wine, lemon juice, silken tofu, rosemary, salt and pepper to a blender and blitz together, then add to the pan with the garlic and mushrooms. If the sauce is a little thick, you can add some water or soya milk to thin it out.

4. Cook the pasta according to the packet instructions.

5. Drain the pasta and serve topped with the mushroom sauce and scatter with the chopped walnuts.

Recipes: Week 2

N.B. Each meal serves two people
unless otherwise stated.

SHOPPING LIST

Dairy alternatives

- [ ] 250g pot coconut yoghurt (some to be used next week so keep in fridge!)
- [ ] 1 litre almond milk
- [ ] 1 litre hazelnut milk

Fruit and vegetables

- [ ] 3 white onions
- [ ] 6 red onions
- [ ] 1 sweet potato
- [ ] 6 spring onions
- [ ] 2 red peppers and 1 pepper of your choice
- [ ] 3 small pak choi (or 1-2 big ones!)
- [ ] 100g sugar snap peas
- [ ] 1 cauliflower
- [ ] 1 beetroot
- [ ] 3 medium avocados
- [ ] 2 bunches asparagus
- [ ] 4 tomatoes
- [ ] 100g cherry tomatoes
- [ ] 200g kale
- [ ] 3 celery sticks
- [ ] ½ cucumber
- [ ] 2 aubergines
- [ ] 2 large fennel bulbs
- [ ] 100g artichoke hearts (from the deli section)
- [ ] 200g wild mushrooms
- [ ] 80g pomegranate seeds (or leftovers from week 1)
- [ ] 2 courgettes
- [ ] 1 broccoli head
- [ ] 1 x 198g tin pineapple chunks
- [ ] 2 limes
- [ ] 1 dessert apple
- [ ] 6 lemons
- [ ] 2 cooking apples
- [ ] 350g frozen mixed berries
- [ ] 4 small-medium bananas
- [ ] 4 dried apricots
- [ ] 30g blueberries

Carbohydrate staples

- [ ] 2 burger buns/ bread rolls
- [ ] 2 flatbreads
- [ ] 110g fresh breadcrumbs*

Dried store foods

- [ ] 1 x 400g tin coconut milk
- [ ] 2 x 400g tins butter beans
- [ ] 3 x 400g tins chickpeas
- [ ] 1 x 198g tin sweetcorn
- [ ] 1 x 400g tin chopped tomatoes
- [ ] 1 x 200g tin haricot beans
- [ ] 1 x 400g tin cannellini beans

Other

- [ ] 200g ready-cooked firm tofu
- [ ] 50g dried cranberries
- [ ] 250g pine nuts
- [ ] 150g sundried tomatoes
- [ ] 125g cacao nibs
- [ ] 30g freeze-dried raspberries (if you prefer, you can use other dried fruits)

- [ ] 50g dessicated coconut
- [ ] 2 lemongrass sticks

Fresh herbs

- [ ] Mint**
- [ ] Coriander**
- [ ] Chives
- [ ] Parsley**
- [ ] Dill

*Instead of buying breadcrumbs, you can make some (see page 160 for recipe)

**You may not need to buy these if you have leftovers from last week.

MENU

	Breakfast	Lunch	Dinner
Saturday	Quinoa granola with dried raspberries and cacao nibs	Broad bean, asparagus and mint tartine	A Lebanese feast: imam, hummus, flatbread and a nutty kale salad
Sunday	Pancakes with stewed autumn fruits and coconut yoghurt	Fennel and white bean soup	Caponata-inspired spaghetti
Monday	Chia pudding with coconut, pomegranate and pistachios	Artichoke and broad bean salad with a tahini dressing	Red Thai butter bean curry with wild rice
Tuesday	Berry blast smoothie	Rainbow wild rice salad with a tangy dressing	Korean quinoa bowls

	Breakfast	Lunch	Dinner
Wednesday	Multi-grain porridge	Nutty quinoa salad with fresh veggies and mustard vinaigrette	'Shepherd-less' pie with sweet potato mash
Thursday	Smashed avocado and spiced chickpeas on toast	Fennel, white bean and courgetti salad with tahini dressing	Beetroot sliders
Friday	Apricot, blueberry and hazelnut bircher muesli	Leftover beetroot sliders with buckwheat tabbouleh	Lemon and pea risotto with roasted asparagus spears

BREAKFAST

Quinoa granola with dried raspberries and cacao nibs

Makes enough for approx. 10 servings. Under 450 calories per serving

If you are a chocoholic, this granola will be your idea of breakfast heaven. The granola also keeps really well – you can store it in a sealed container at room temperature for about a month – and is useful for other breakfasts, and as a snack! I like mine on its own, but you could also have it with soya milk or a nut milk of your choice.

180g rolled oats	1 tsp ground cinnamon
140g quinoa	¼ tsp salt
100g flaked almonds	30g freeze-dried raspberries (if
60g chia seeds	you prefer, you can use other
150ml maple syrup	dried fruits)
150ml melted coconut oil	125g cacao nibs

1. Preheat the oven to 170°C/150°C fan/325°F/gas mark 3 and line a large baking sheet with baking parchment.

2. In a large bowl, mix together the oats, quinoa, almonds and chia seeds.

3. In a separate bowl, whisk together the maple syrup, coconut oil, cinnamon and salt.

4. Pour the wet ingredients over the dry and stir until all the dry ingredients are coated. Spread the granola mixture into an even layer over the baking sheet and bake for 40 minutes, turning regularly so that the mixture doesn't burn.

5. Remove from the oven. With a spatula, press the mixture down gently, to make sure 'clusters' of the granola form, then let it cool completely.

6. Toss in the freeze-dried raspberries and cacao nibs and transfer to an airtight container until needed.

LUNCH

Broad bean, asparagus and mint tartine

Under 550 calories

This makes a very pretty lunch. A tartine is a French open sandwich – if you're hungry, use extra slices of toast to make closed sandwiches.

4 slices of sourdough, toasted
Mint leaves, to serve

FOR THE BROAD BEAN
PURÉE
150g frozen broad beans
1 white onion, diced
½ tbsp olive oil

1 garlic clove, crushed
Zest and juice of 1 lemon
Salt and pepper, to taste

FOR THE ROASTED
ASPARAGUS SPEARS
1 bunch of asparagus
Drizzle of balsamic glaze

1. Preheat the oven to 180°C/160°C fan/350°F/gas mark 4.

2. First make the broad bean purée. Simmer the beans in a pan of boiling water for 5 minutes until tender. Drain.

3. In a pan over a medium heat, fry the onion in the olive oil for about 5 minutes, until soft. Add the garlic and cook for 2 minutes until fragrant and soft. Tip into a blender along with the broad beans, lemon zest and juice and blitz until smooth. Season with salt and pepper to taste.

4. Next, roast the asparagus. Spread the asparagus out over a baking tray and drizzle with the balsamic glaze, then roast in the oven for 10 minutes, until soft and slightly caramelised.

5. Toast the sourdough, spread with the broad bean purée, pile with the asparagus and tear over the mint leaves.

DINNER

A Lebanese feast: imam, hummus, flatbread and a nutty kale salad

Under 900 calories (for a lower-calorie meal, you could reduce the hummus by half and leave out the flatbread – under 700 calories)

The aubergine has been called the 'poor man's meat' – probably because it is a great meat alternative! The 'imam' recipe can be served hot or cold, so you can always make extra and keep it for lunches.

FOR THE IMAM
1 aubergine
1 tbsp olive oil
1 small red onion, diced
1 garlic clove, minced
½ tbsp dried oregano
½ tbsp Moroccan spice mix (or cinnamon if you struggle to buy this!)
2 large tomatoes, diced
Salt and pepper, to taste

FOR THE NUTTY KALE SALAD
200g kale, tough stalks removed
Juice of 1 lemon
1 tbsp olive oil
30g flaked almonds
30g hazelnuts
50g dried cranberries

FOR THE CARAMELISED RED ONION HUMMUS
1 red onion, sliced thinly
1½ tbsp olive oil
1 tbsp dark muscovado sugar
1½ tbsp balsamic vinegar
1 x 400g tin chickpeas, drained and rinsed
Juice of 1 lemon
2 tsp tahini
2 tsp Moroccan spice mix
3 tbsp water
Small handful of flat-leaf parsley

TO SERVE
2 flatbreads

Saturday

1. Preheat the oven to 180°C/160°C fan/350°F/gas mark 4.
   Line a baking tray with baking parchment.

2. Start by making the imam. Cut the aubergine in half
   lengthways, then score the flesh deeply (making sure you do
   not cut through the skin). Drizzle each half aubergine with ½
   a tablespoon of olive oil and a pinch of salt.

3. Lay the aubergine cut-side down on the baking tray and roast
   in the oven for 20 minutes, until soft.

4. While the aubergine is roasting, cook the stuffing for the
   imam. In a frying pan on a medium heat, heat the remaining
   ½ tablespoon of olive oil, then add the red onion and garlic.
   Fry for about 5 minutes until aromatic. Add the herbs and
   spices and cook for another minute until well mixed.

5. Add the tomatoes and cook gently for another 10 minutes,
   stirring to make sure the mixture doesn't 'catch' on the
   bottom of the pan.

6. Remove the aubergines from the oven and turn each over
   gently, being careful not to rip the skins. Scoop out the
   scored flesh (do not throw away the skins) and stir it into the
   stuffing mixture in the frying pan.

7. Layer the stuffing inside the aubergine skins and return to the
   oven to bake for another 10 minutes, until browned slightly
   on top. Heat the flatbreads through in the oven with the
   imam for the final few minutes of cooking.

8. Meanwhile, make the kale salad. Tear the kale leaves into small pieces and add to a serving bowl, then drizzle over the lemon juice and olive oil and massage into the leaves. Toast the nuts and cranberries in a dry frying pan for about 5 minutes. Make sure the nuts don't burn – they turn from under-done to burnt very quickly! When ready, leave to cool for a minute and then scatter over the kale.

9. To make the hummus, start by caramelising the onion. In a frying pan, cook the onion in 1 tablespoon of olive oil until soft – about 5 minutes. Add the sugar and balsamic vinegar, and cook for another 3 minutes, until caramelised.

10. Add the chickpeas, the rest of the olive oil, lemon juice, tahini and Moroccan spice mix to a blender and blitz until completely smooth. Add the water, a small amount at a time, until you reach the desired consistency. Add salt and pepper to taste. Scoop from the blender into a serving bowl and top with caramelised red onion and parsley.

11. Serve the imam with the kale salad, hummus and the warmed flatbreads for dipping.

BREAKFAST

Pancakes with stewed autumn fruits and coconut yoghurt

Under 550 calories

Often people think pancakes are really unhealthy – and they are if you load them with sugar and syrups! But here, with lots of fruit, they make a filling and healthier alternative to many other pancakes out there.

FOR THE PANCAKES
70g plain flour
1 tsp baking powder
¼ tsp salt
150ml almond milk
1 tbsp maple syrup
½ tsp vanilla extract
2 tbsp vegan butter, softened,
    plus extra for cooking

FOR THE STEWED FRUIT
2 tbsp vegan butter
2 tbsp dark muscovado sugar
2 cooking apples, peeled, cored
    and diced
100g frozen mixed berries
1 tsp ground cinnamon

TO SERVE
2 tbsp coconut yoghurt
Maple syrup

1. First make the stewed fruit. Put the vegan butter and sugar in a saucepan over a low heat and melt together. Cook for 3 minutes until the mixture turns a light caramel.

2. Stir in the diced apples, berries and cinnamon, then cover the pan and leave to stew for 10 minutes. If the mixture starts to dry out, add some water, a few tablespoons at a time.

3. Meanwhile, prepare the pancakes. Place the dry ingredients in a bowl and stir to combine. Then add all the wet ingredients, including the butter, and mix until smooth. To get the lumps out, it may be best to use a balloon whisk.

4. Heat some vegan butter in a shallow frying pan over a medium heat. Pour a heaped spoonful of pancake batter onto the hot pan and cook until bubbles form. Then flip and cook the other side. Keep warm while you cook another three pancakes in the same way.

5. When you have cooked all four pancakes, serve two each on two plates with the stewed fruit, coconut yoghurt and a drizzle of maple syrup.

LUNCH

Fennel and white bean soup

Under 300 calories

It can be difficult to spread your protein evenly throughout the day, but the beans in this soup certainly make that easier. I blend the soup to make it smooth, but it is also delicious chunky, if you prefer.

2 tbsp olive oil
1 white onion, chopped
1 large fennel bulb, thinly
   sliced (fronds trimmed and
   reserved)
1 garlic clove, finely diced
½ x 400g tin cannellini beans,
   drained and rinsed (decant
   the other half into a bowl,
   cover it and keep in the
   fridge for lunch on Thursday)

350ml vegetable stock, made
   from 1 stock cube
Salt and pepper, to taste

TO SERVE
2 tbsp coconut yoghurt
Fronds from the fennel bulb,
   chopped
Small bunch of chives, chopped

1. In a saucepan over a medium heat, heat the olive oil and cook the onion until softened, 3–4 minutes.

2. Turn down the heat to low, then add the fennel and garlic and cook until very soft, about 20 minutes.

3. Add the beans and stock, bring to the boil and simmer for 10 minutes. Season with salt and pepper, then blitz with a hand-held blender in the pan or transfer to a blender until smooth.

4. Serve with a swirl of coconut yoghurt, and garnish with the chopped fennel fronds and chives.

DINNER

Caponata-inspired spaghetti

Under 600 calories

Caponata is a Sicilian dish made with aubergines and capers in a sweet-and-sour sauce. Here you get the flavours of caponata in a one-pot spaghetti recipe, and it really couldn't be easier to make.

1 tbsp olive oil

1 aubergine, cut into small chunks

1 tbsp dried oregano

150g wholewheat spaghetti

1 x 400g tin chopped tomatoes

1 tbsp capers

1 red onion, diced

1 garlic clove, diced

300ml vegetable stock, made from 1 stock cube

Salt and pepper, to taste

50g flaked almonds

Small handful of flat-leaf parsley, finely chopped (stalks and leaves), to serve

1. Start by frying the aubergine. Put the olive oil into a deep saucepan (as you'll be using this pan to cook the pasta) and add the aubergine and oregano. Fry for about 5 minutes, until the aubergine starts to turn golden.

2. Add all the remaining ingredients, except the almonds and parsley, to the pan and leave to bubble away for 10–12 minutes, stirring regularly, until the pasta is al dente. At this stage, the sauce should be lovely and thick.

3. In a separate frying pan, toast the almonds by dry-frying them for about 5 minutes over a low heat, stirring constantly. They will burn quickly so make sure you watch them!

4. Serve the spaghetti and sauce topped with chopped parsley and almonds.

Get ahead

You can prepare the chia seeds for breakfast tomorrow now if you like; this should only take a few minutes and you can do this while the pasta is bubbling away and the sauce thickens.

BREAKFAST

Chia pudding with coconut, pomegranate and pistachios

Under 500 calories

Chia puddings make good breakfasts as they can be prepared the night before, saving you valuable time in the mornings. But if you forget to do it the night before, they can also be ready in just half an hour.

60g chia seeds	500ml almond milk
2 tsp agave nectar	50g dessicated coconut
2 tsp vanilla extract	50g pistachio nuts
2 tbsp coconut yoghurt	80g pomegranate seeds

1. Divide the chia seeds, agave, vanilla extract and yoghurt among two bowls.

2. Pour in the milk and stir everything together.

3. Leave to stand for 15 minutes, then stir again.

4. Put the bowls in the fridge overnight for the next morning, or set aside while you get ready for the day ahead. The chia seeds will expand to absorb all the liquid and form a jellylike consistency in about half an hour.

5. Just before serving, toast the dessicated coconut and pistachios in a dry frying pan over a low-to-medium heat for about 5 minutes, stirring constantly. Make sure the nuts don't burn – they should smell lovely and aromatic when cooked.

6. Take the bowls of chia pudding out of the fridge and top with the nuts and pomegranate seeds.

LUNCH

Artichoke and broad bean salad with a tahini dressing

Under 400 calories

The dressing for this salad, thanks to the addition of lemon juice, is really full of flavour. You can always make more than you need and keep it in the fridge for use in other salads, too – just be aware that it will thicken up when it is chilled.

FOR THE SALAD
100g barley
200g broad beans, fresh or
    frozen
100g artichoke hearts, sliced
Small bunch of mint, chopped
    finely

Small bunch of parsley,
    chopped finely

FOR THE TAHINI DRESSING
2 tsp tahini
4 tsp olive oil
Salt and pepper, to taste
Juice of 1 lemon

1. First make the dressing. Stir together all the ingredients, then transfer half of the dressing to a covered jug or sealed container and pop in the fridge for lunch on Thursday.

2. Cook the barley according to the packet instructions.

3. Boil the broad beans in a pan of boiling water for about 3 minutes until cooked through (you will need to boil for longer if they are frozen than if they are fresh).

4. Combine the barley, beans, artichoke hearts and herbs in a serving bowl and toss with the dressing just before serving.

DINNER

Red Thai butter bean curry with wild rice

Under 800 calories

This is a good alternative to traditional red Thai chicken curry, just make sure you don't add the beans too early – otherwise they will fall apart.

200g wild rice

1 tbsp olive oil

2 garlic cloves, minced

2 spring onions, thinly sliced

Thumb-sized piece of fresh
    root ginger, finely grated

1 red pepper, deseeded and
    diced

3 tbsp red Thai curry paste

1 x 400g tin coconut milk

3 small pak choi (or 1-2 big
    ones!), thinly sliced

1 x 400g tin butter beans,
    drained and rinsed

Handful of coriander, chopped,
    to serve

2 tbsp coconut yoghurt,
    to serve

1. Cook the wild rice according to the packet instructions.

2. While the wild rice is cooking, start the curry. Heat the olive oil in a wok over a medium heat and sweat down the garlic, onions, ginger and red pepper. This should take about 5 minutes.

3. When the vegetables in the wok are soft, add the red Thai curry paste and stir to coat, cooking for another few minutes just to heat through.

4. Pour in the coconut milk and cook with the lid off for about 10 minutes, until the sauce has started to thicken.

5. Add the pak choi and butter beans and heat through, making sure you don't stir the curry too much to avoid breaking up the butter beans.

6. Save half of the rice for lunch tomorrow, then divide the remaining rice among two bowls. Serve the curry on top of the rice, each sprinkled with coriander and topped with coconut yoghurt.

BREAKFAST

Berry blast smoothie

Under 500 calories

Frozen fruit is perfect for smoothies; not only is it often cheaper than fresh fruit, but it is available year round and makes the smoothie lovely and cold, too. If you use fresh fruit instead, add a few ice cubes when blending or serve the smoothie over ice.

600ml hazelnut milk	2 scoops of soya protein
2 bananas	powder
250g frozen mixed berries	40g bran flakes

1. Combine all the ingredients in a blender and blitz until smooth and thoroughly mixed.

2. Divide among two glasses.

LUNCH

Rainbow wild rice salad with a tangy dressing

Under 500 calories

This lunch is unbelievably colourful. We eat with all our senses, eyes included, so having a colourful, pretty meal makes it really appetizing. This is also great with the dressing from Monday's lunch.

FOR THE WILD RICE SALAD
100g sugar snap peas
100g garden peas
1 small red onion, thinly sliced
1 x 198g tin sweetcorn, drained
1 x 400g tin chickpeas, drained
  and rinsed
Cooked wild rice (from last
  night's dinner)

Handful of coriander leaves,
  chopped

FOR THE DRESSING
Zest and juice of 1 lime
2 tsp agave nectar
½ tsp chilli flakes (or more if
  you're feeling brave!)

1. Whisk all the dressing ingredients together and set aside.

2. Blanch the sugar snap peas and garden peas in a pan of boiling water for about 3 minutes, until softened, then drain and rinse under cold water (this stops them cooking any further and keeps them nice and bright green).

3. Mix together the blanched vegetables, onion, sweetcorn, chickpeas and rice in a large bowl, then toss with the dressing and coriander. If you are making this to take to work, keep the dressing on the side until you are ready to eat it.

DINNER

Korean quinoa bowls

Under 500 calories without the sauce; under 600 calories with ¼ of the BBQ sauce

Don't be put off by the long list of ingredients for the BBQ sauce – it is really worth the effort and you'll make a big batch, which is great for many other recipes! However, if you're particularly tight for time, you could always buy a bottle of it.

FOR THE BBQ SAUCE
125ml ketchup
125ml rice vinegar
60ml soy sauce
1½ tbsp sugar
1 tbsp sesame seeds
2 tsp yellow miso
1 tsp sriracha
¼ tsp black pepper
2 spring onions, thinly sliced
1 garlic clove, minced
1 x 2½cm piece of root ginger, grated
2 tsp olive oil

FOR THE BOWL
240g quinoa
1 tbsp olive oil
½ head cauliflower, cut into small florets
1 red pepper, deseeded and diced
2 spring onions, cut into small discs
200g ready-cooked firm tofu
1 x 198g tin pineapple chunks
½ tsp chilli flakes

1. To make the sauce, whisk together all the ingredients except the sesame oil in a pan over a medium heat. Bring to a simmer, whisking all the time. Leave to simmer for 15 minutes, whisking regularly, until a thick paste forms, before removing from the heat and adding the sesame oil. Set aside. You will make a large amount of the sauce, so pour some into a sterilised bottle (see page 46) for use in Friday's dinner too.

2. Cook the quinoa according to the packet instructions.

3. Heat the olive oil in a wok or saucepan over a medium heat. Add the cauliflower, pepper and spring onions. Stir-fry until the pepper and spring onions are softened and the cauliflower is cooked through but still has some 'bite' – about 15 minutes.

4. Tip the tofu into a clean tea towel and squeeze to remove as much water as possible, then add this to the pan and heat through.

5. Save half the quinoa for tomorrow's lunch. To serve, layer the bowl with quinoa on the bottom, then the veggies, then the tofu and top with a generous drizzle of the BBQ sauce.

BREAKFAST

Multi-grain porridge

Under 600 calories without toppings

There's lots of confusion around the difference between 'wholegrain' and 'multi-grain.' Multi just means that it contains more than one grain, whereas wholegrain means that it contains the rusk of the grain (the outside shell, which is high in fibre). The toppings are up to you – personally I like it with jam and coconut flakes.

50g rolled oats
50g barley
50g quinoa
50g linseeds
2 bananas, sliced
350ml almond milk

TO SERVE (OPTIONAL)
Maple syrup or chia jam

---

1. Put all the ingredients into a saucepan over a medium heat and heat gently, stirring constantly, until all the liquid is absorbed and the porridge is really creamy. This should take 4–5 minutes.

2. Serve in two bowls, topped with your choice of maple syrup or chia jam (made in week 1), and scattered with coconut flakes.

LUNCH

Nutty quinoa salad with fresh veggies and mustard vinaigrette

Under 600 calories

This salad contains a brilliant variety of textures – from the soft avocado to the crunchy nuts. You will make more vinaigrette than you need, so store it in a sterilised bottle (see page 46) in the fridge for later use, where it will keep for a few weeks. If you are making this ahead of time and taking it to work for lunch, I'd recommend keeping the dressing separate and adding it just before eating, so the nuts keep their crunch.

FOR THE SALAD
Cooked quinoa (leftover from last night's dinner)
1 avocado, halved, stoned, peeled and cut into small chunks
100g cherry tomatoes, halved
1 pepper (red, orange or yellow), deseeded and diced
¼ cucumber, cut into small chunks
Small bunch of coriander, chopped

Small bunch of flat-leaf parsley, chopped
50g pine nuts, toasted
50g flaked almonds
Salt and pepper, to taste

FOR THE VINAIGRETTE
½ tsp English mustard
20ml balsamic vinegar
60ml olive oil

1. To make the vinaigrette, whisk the mustard and vinegar to a paste. Slowly add the olive oil, a little bit at a time, so that the oil emulsifies, giving you a smooth dressing.

2. In a serving bowl, combine the quinoa, avocado, cherry tomatoes, pepper, cucumber and chopped herbs.

3. Season to taste, and sprinkle over the pine nuts and almonds.

4. Serve drizzled with the vinaigrette.

DINNER

'Shepherd-less' pie with sweet potato mash

Under 600 calories

This recipe is another great one for converting your meat-loving friends to a vegan diet. You get so much flavour from the mushrooms, sundried tomatoes and herbs that you will definitely not miss the meat. You also get a lovely golden colour and crunch from the breadcrumb topping.

1 tbsp olive oil
1 red onion, diced
3 garlic cloves, minced
1 celery stick, finely chopped
200g wild mushrooms, cut into strips
150g sundried tomatoes
4 tsp dried rosemary
1 tbsp plain flour

150ml vegetable stock, made from 1 stock cube
1 x 200g tin haricot beans, drained and rinsed
1 sweet potato, peeled and cut into chunks
1 tbsp vegan butter
60g breadcrumbs
Salt and pepper, to taste

1. Preheat the oven to 200°C/180°C fan/400°F/gas mark 6.

2. In a large saucepan, heat the olive oil, then add the red onion, garlic and celery. Sweat for about 10 minutes until very soft.

3. Add the mushrooms and cook for a further 10 minutes.

4. Add the sundried tomatoes and rosemary to the saucepan and stir to combine.

5. Add the plain flour to the vegetable stock and stir into a thick paste, then add to the saucepan. Add the beans. Bubble for a few minutes until the sauce is thick and all the ingredients are well combined, then tip the mixture into an ovenproof dish.

6. To make the mashed potato, boil the sweet potato for about 10 minutes, then mash until smooth with the vegan butter, liberal amounts of pepper and a little salt.

7. Tip the mash on top of the vegetable-bean mix and spread out to completely cover.

8. Sprinkle the top with breadcrumbs and bake for 10 minutes, until piping hot throughout and the crumb topping is golden.

BREAKFAST

Smashed avocado and spiced chickpeas on toast

Under 600 calories

This breakfast requires a little bit more preparation than the others, as you need to toast the chickpeas. If you are not a morning person and therefore might struggle with this, you can use the chickpeas untoasted, as tinned chickpeas are already cooked.

FOR THE SMASHED AVOCADO
1 avocado, halved, stoned and
    peeled
Juice of 1 lime
1 tbsp olive oil
Salt, pepper and Tabasco sauce,
    to taste

FOR THE CHICKPEAS
2 tbsp olive oil
3 tsp Moroccan spice mix
1 x 400g tin chickpeas, drained

TO SERVE
2 slices of sourdough

1. In a bowl, mash the avocado, lime juice, olive oil, salt, pepper and Tabasco to taste.

2. Heat a saucepan on a medium-high heat, add the olive oil and spices, and heat for 1 minute.

3. Add the chickpeas to the hot spices and toss to coat. Cook for another minute until the chickpeas are heated through.

4. Toast the sourdough, then top with the mashed avocado and spiced chickpeas.

LUNCH

Fennel, white bean and courgetti salad with tahini dressing

Under 400 calories

'Spiralised' vegetables became very popular as a pasta alternative. However, there is nothing wrong with carbohydrates (see page 18 for information about carbohydrates), and you should only eat spiralised vegetables if you like them, not to avoid carbs! If you don't have a spiraliser, you can just use a peeler – you'll end up with ribbons rather than noodle shapes but the effect is the same.

50g flaked almonds
2 courgettes
1 x 200g tin cannellini beans, drained and rinsed
1 fennel bulb, very thinly sliced

Tahini dressing (leftover from Monday's lunch)
Small bunch of dill, finely chopped

---

1. In a dry frying pan over a low heat, toast the almonds for about 5 minutes, stirring constantly. They will burn quickly so make sure you watch them! Set aside.

2. Spiralise the courgettes. If you don't have a spiraliser, you can use a peeler to make 'ribbons'.

3. Mix the beans and fennel with the courgetti.

4. Toss the courgetti, beans and fennel with the tahini dressing and sprinkle over the toasted nuts and chopped dill.

DINNER

Beetroot sliders

Under 600 calories without sauce; under 700 calories with ½ leftover sauce

Sliders are mini burgers; here I've used them as a main course but they also make a great canapé and leftovers will make a useful lunch tomorrow. As well as making these tonight, you will need to prepare Friday's breakfast.

FOR THE BURGERS
1 red onion, diced
1 garlic clove, diced
2 tbsp olive oil, plus extra to fry
    the patties
1 beetroot, grated
1 dessert apple, grated
½ cauliflower head, grated
½ tsp chilli flakes
1 x 400g tin butter beans,
    drained and rinsed
1 tbsp horseradish sauce

1 tbsp peanut butter
50g breadcrumbs (see page
    160 to make your own)
Salt and pepper, to taste

TO SERVE
2 burger buns, sliced
1 avocado, halved, stoned,
    peeled and sliced
BBQ sauce (from Tuesday's
    dinner)

1. Cook the onion and garlic together in the olive oil in a large pan over a medium heat until soft.

2. Add the rest of the ingredients and cook until all liquid has cooked, 5–10 minutes.

3. Leave the mixture to cool, then take handfuls of the mixture, shape them into the size of a golf ball and flatten to make patties. You will have more than you need at this stage – you should allow two per person for dinner, and two per person for lunch tomorrow. You can also freeze the raw mixture at this stage and defrost the patties at a later date for another meal.

4. Take eight patties and fry them in a little oil in a non-stick pan for about 5 minutes on each side until brown on both sides. You may need to do this in batches. Set half aside for lunch tomorrow.

5. Layer the sliders with the BBQ sauce and sliced avo in a burger bun. Save the other four sliders for lunch tomorrow!

Get ahead

You need to prepare the oats tonight and pop them in the fridge for tomorrow morning's breakfast – see step 1 of the recipe.

BREAKFAST

Apricot, blueberry and hazelnut bircher muesli

Under 600 calories

Bircher muesli is also known as 'overnight oats'. When you leave oats overnight in liquid, they will expand and absorb all the moisture, giving you a lovely creamy texture similar to porridge. You can really taste the flavour of the hazelnut milk in this recipe.

80g rolled oats	30g hazelnuts
400ml hazelnut milk	30g flaked almonds
2 tbsp maple syrup	30g blueberries
1 tsp vanilla extract	4 dried apricots, diced

1. Combine the oats, hazelnut milk, maple syrup and vanilla extract in a large bowl, cover and leave in the fridge overnight.

2. In the morning, toast the hazelnuts and flaked almonds in a dry frying pan for about 3 minutes, until fragrant, stirring constantly. They will burn quickly so make sure you watch them!

3. Divide the oat mix among two bowls and top with toasted nuts and fruits to serve.

LUNCH

Leftover beetroot sliders with buckwheat tabbouleh

Under 800 calories

Tabbouleh is a traditional Levantine dish. It is normally made with bulgur wheat, but here I've used buckwheat to give it a new twist.

200g buckwheat

2 tomatoes, diced

¼ cucumber, diced

Small handful of parsley, finely chopped

1 garlic clove, crushed

1½ tbsp olive oil

Zest and juice of 1 lemon

4 beetroot sliders (from yesterday's dinner)

Salt and pepper, to taste

1. Cook the buckwheat according to the packet instructions.

2. Mix the tomatoes, cucumber and parsley together in a bowl.

3. Whisk the garlic clove, olive oil, lemon juice and zest together in a small bowl, then drizzle it over the tabbouleh. Serve topped with the beetroot sliders.

DINNER

Lemon and pea risotto with roasted asparagus spears

Under 550 calories

Blending the onion and celery gives this risotto a really smooth consistency but with plenty of flavour. If you don't have a blender, just finely chop the onions and celery.

1 white onion, peeled and roughly chopped

2 celery sticks, roughly chopped

1½ tbsp olive oil

175g risotto rice

500ml vegetable stock, made from 1 stock cube

1 bunch of asparagus spears

Balsamic vinegar, for drizzling

150g frozen garden peas

Zest and juice of 1 lemon

Salt and pepper, to taste

1. Preheat the oven to 180°C/160°C fan/350°F/gas mark 4.

2. Put the onion in a blender with the celery and blitz until finely chopped. You may need to stop the blender and scrape down the sides with a spatula a few times during blending.

3. Put ½ tablespoon of the olive oil in a saucepan with the blended celery and onion mix, and fry for about 5 minutes over a low heat until soft.

4. Remove the celery-onion blend from the pan and set aside.

5. Using the same pan, heat ½ tablespoon of olive oil, before adding the risotto rice. Stir the grains to coat them thoroughly in the oil and fry until translucent (less than 1 minute), then slowly add the stock, a small amount at a time, until all the liquid is absorbed. If you do this too quickly the risotto will be very stodgy – it should take at least 15 minutes.

6. Meanwhile, put the asparagus on a baking tray with the remaining olive oil and drizzle with balsamic vinegar. Roast the asparagus for 10–15 minutes, until softened but still with some 'bite'.

7. While the risotto is cooking, boil the peas for a few minutes until soft. Blend about two-thirds of the peas with the lemon juice and zest, setting aside the other third.

8. When the risotto has finished cooking, stir through the green pea purée, sprinkle the reserved peas over and place half the asparagus spears on top. (Reserve the remaining asparagus spears for tomorrow's lunch in a pot in the fridge.) Serve immediately.

Recipes: Week 3

N.B. Each meal serves two people
unless otherwise stated.

SHOPPING LIST

Dairy alternatives

☐ 1 litre hazelnut milk

☐ 1 litre almond milk

Fruit and vegetables

☐ 4 red onions

☐ 1 white onion

☐ 1 large potato

☐ 1 sweet potato

☐ 6 spring onions

☐ 600g cherry tomatoes

☐ 2 small cucumbers

☐ 4 avocados

☐ 300g spinach

☐ 3 red peppers

☐ 4 Romano peppers

☐ 1 little gem lettuce

☐ 125g bag of rocket

☐ 150g sundried tomatoes

☐ 150g artichoke hearts

☐ 3 aubergines

☐ 150g chestnut mushrooms

☐ 3 carrots

☐ 1 beetroot

☐ 1 courgette

☐ 100g green beans

☐ 4 plum tomatoes

☐ 1 very small red cabbage

☐ 4 limes

☐ 4 lemons

☐ 130g fresh pineapple chunks

☐ 6 plums

☐ 4 bananas

☐ 2 dessert apples

☐ 1 small mango

☐ 100g raspberries

☐ 100g strawberries

Dried store foods

- [ ] 2 x 400ml tins reduced-fat coconut milk
- [ ] 2 x 400g tins chickpeas
- [ ] 1 x 400g tin butter beans
- [ ] 1 x 227g tin chopped tomatoes
- [ ] 200g ready-to-eat quinoa lentil mix
- [ ] 110g preserved lemon

Other

- [ ] 400ml orange juice
- [ ] 3 sheets sushi nori
- [ ] Wasabi paste
- [ ] Pickled ginger
- [ ] 600g tempeh (tofu is OK if you can't find any tempeh!)

- [ ] 70g pine nuts (leftover from last week)
- [ ] 50g dessicated coconut
- [ ] 30g sultanas
- [ ] 50g dried cranberries (leftover from week 2)

Fresh herbs

- [ ] Coriander*
- [ ] Mint*
- [ ] Parsley*
- [ ] Dill*
- [ ] Basil

*You may not need to buy these if you have leftovers from previous weeks.

MENU

	Breakfast	Lunch	Dinner
Saturday	Raw date, pecan and walnut breakfast bars	Borscht	Aubergine katsu curry
Sunday	Rösti topped with rocket and mashed avo	Hot aubergine pockets	Tempeh kebabs with a peanut dipping sauce
Monday	Layered summer fruit parfait with coconut yoghurt and granola	Sourdough fattoush with butter beans	Sweet potato and chickpea curry with a spiced tomato salad
Tuesday	Cacao, date and banana smoothie	Indian-spiced tomato and white bean salad	Quinoa bowl – harissa roasted aubergine, garlic mushrooms, spinach and hummus

	Breakfast	Lunch	Dinner
Wednesday	Apple and ginger bircher muesli	Gado-gado with quinoa	Vegan quinoa sushi
Thursday	Tropical popical smoothie	Mango, tomato and basil salad	Spinach crepes with a pepper filling
Friday	Porridge with vanilla poached plums	Turkish tomato salad with coconut haydari	Quinoa-stuffed peppers with Moroccan flavours

BREAKFAST

Raw date, pecan and walnut breakfast bars

Makes 10. Under 300 calories per bar

These bars don't need cooking; instead you just combine the ingredients and press together. They are so easy to make and the mixture will make 10 bars, so put the rest into an airtight container and keep for on-the-go breakfasts and snacks! You can either keep them in the fridge for one week or in the freezer for a month or two.

220g pitted medjool dates	140g rolled oats
85ml maple syrup	50g pecans, chopped
65g peanut butter	90g walnuts, chopped
2 tsp vanilla extract	

1. Line a 20 x 20cm square baking tin with baking parchment.

2. Blitz the dates in a food processor with the maple syrup, peanut butter and vanilla extract.

3. In a shallow dry frying pan over a low heat, toast the oats for about 10 minutes, stirring regularly. Add the nuts for the last few minutes, stirring until they turn brown.

4. Place the toasted oats and nuts in a large mixing bowl and pour over the wet date and peanut butter mixture. Mix until thoroughly combined.

5. Transfer the mixture into the baking dish and press down firmly.

6. Chill the breakfast bars in a freezer for 20 minutes before cutting into 10 bars.

LUNCH

Borscht

Under 300 calories

Borscht is a traditional eastern European soup, made from beetroot. It is very vibrant and has a lovely, earthy taste from the beetroot. I blend this soup, but you can have it chunky if you prefer.

---

1 red onion, sliced

1 carrot, sliced

1 beetroot, sliced

1 garlic clove, finely chopped

½ x 400g tin chopped
   tomatoes

600ml vegetable stock

1 tbsp tomato purée

1 tsp dark muscovado sugar

½ very small red cabbage, sliced

TO SERVE

Dill leaves, chopped

Salt and pepper, to taste

---

1. In a large pan, stir together all the ingredients and simmer over a low heat for 30 minutes, until all the vegetables are very soft. Keep the pan covered as you do this, so you don't lose too much moisture.

2. Blitz with a hand-held blender in the pan or transfer to a blender and whiz until smooth. Season well and serve topped with the chopped dill.

DINNER

Aubergine katsu curry

Under 750 calories

Traditional katsu curries are made from a smooth, silky sauce poured over a breaded chicken fillet; here the chicken is substituted with large pieces of aubergine 'steaks' to make a hearty vegan alternative. If you have friends over who are not vegan, or are getting into veganism for the first time, this dish is a really good choice.

FOR THE CRISPY AUBERGINE
2 aubergines
100ml almond milk
100g dried breadcrumbs
2 tbsp olive oil
Salt and pepper, to taste

FOR THE CURRY SAUCE
1 tbsp olive oil
½ white onion, peeled and diced (save the other half for dinner on Monday)
3 garlic cloves, peeled and finely chopped
1 carrot, peeled and finely chopped
1 tbsp plain flour
½ tbsp medium curry powder
1 tsp maple syrup
½ tbsp soy sauce
300ml vegetable stock, made from 1 stock cube
180g rice
Coriander leaves, finely chopped, to serve

1. Preheat the oven to 200°C/180°C fan/400°F/gas mark 6.

2. Prepare the aubergine 'steaks'. First, cut the ends off the aubergines and thinly pare away the skin. Then cut each aubergine lengthways in half, so you have four 'steaks'.

3. Pour the almond milk into a bowl, and add the aubergine steaks, allowing them to soak up some of the liquid.

4. Pour the breadcrumbs onto a plate and season well. Transfer the aubergine steaks to the plate and coat liberally with the breadcrumbs on each side – they should stick to the parts of the aubergine with no skin.

5. To make the curry sauce, heat the olive oil in a pan over a low-to-medium heat. Add the onion, garlic and carrot and sweat for 10–15 minutes, until very soft.

6. Stir in the flour and curry powder, maple syrup and soy sauce.

7. Add the stock, a little bit at a time, stirring constantly (with a small whisk if you have one) to prevent lumps forming.

8. Blitz the sauce with a hand-held blender in the pan or transfer to a blender and whiz until smooth, then return to the saucepan to keep warm.

9. Now cook the aubergine steaks. Heat the olive oil in a frying pan and fry them on both sides until brown and crispy (about 5 minutes), then transfer to the oven and cook for another 20 minutes, until soft.

10. Meanwhile, cook the rice according to the packet instructions.

11. When the aubergine steaks are cooked, save two for lunch tomorrow, and pop them in the fridge, covered.

12. Spoon the rice into a bowl and top with the aubergine steaks, then the sauce, and sprinkle with the chopped coriander.

BREAKFAST

Rösti topped with rocket and mashed avo

Under 600 calories

Rösti is a Swiss dish made of grated potatoes, which are shaped into a patty and fried as a fritter. This gives the potatoes a wonderfully crisp exterior, which is perfect combined with the creamy avocado.

FOR THE RÖSTI
1 large potato
1½ tbsp olive oil
Salt and pepper, to taste

FOR THE MASHED AVOCADO
1 avocado, halved, stoned and
    peeled

Juice of 1 lime
Tabasco sauce, to taste

TO SERVE
150g sundried tomatoes
150g artichoke hearts
Handful of rocket leaves

1. To make the rösti, grate the potato coarsely onto a clean tea towel, then roll the potato in the towel like a sausage, pressing down to remove as much of the moisture as possible.

2. Transfer the potato to a bowl and season with salt and pepper, then divide into two equal portions. Shape each portion into a patty.

3. In a large frying pan, heat the olive oil. Fry the rösti for 5 minutes on each side, until golden brown on the outside and soft on the inside. You may need to do this one at a time, depending on the size of your pan.

4. While the patties cook, mash the avocado with the lime juice, salt, pepper and Tabasco, to taste.

5. Serve the rösti topped with the mashed avocado, and the sundried tomatoes, artichoke hearts and a scattering of rocket leaves.

LUNCH

Hot aubergine pockets

Under 450 calories

This is a delicious, filling sandwich. Reheating the aubergine is really important so it is crispy and hot.

2 wholemeal pittas

2 aubergine 'steaks' from
   Saturday's dinner

Vegan butter, for spreading

½ red cabbage, finely grated

Handful of rocket leaves

1 tsp olive oil

1. First toast the wholemeal pittas.

2. Meanwhile, in a shallow frying pan, reheat the aubergine 'steaks' in a little oil so they are hot through and crispy on the outside.

3. Spread the pittas with vegan butter and stuff with the aubergines, cabbage and rocket leaves.

DINNER

Tempeh kebabs with a peanut dipping sauce

Under 900 calories

Tempeh is similar to tofu, but instead of using only the soya bean curd, it is made by a natural fermentation process that binds the soya beans together. The result is a similar taste to tofu but a very different texture – it is much firmer and so holds together well as a kebab. If you can't find tempeh (it's not sold in all supermarkets) you can use tofu instead, but fry it in a little oil until almost cripsy before skewering so it holds its shape. If you are using wooden kebab sticks here, soak them in water for about 30 minutes first to prevent them burning, or use metal ones. You will need 4 skewers.

FOR THE KEBABS

Red pepper, deseeded and cut into chunks

1 small courgette, sliced into 'coins'

1 red onion, cut into wedges

300g tempeh, cut into 3cm chunks

4 wooden or metal skewers

FOR THE PEANUT DIPPING SAUCE

½ tbsp olive oil

80g peanuts

1 garlic clove, minced

1 tsp chilli flakes

1 tsp turmeric

1 tsp soy sauce

Juice of 1 lime

2 tsp water

TO SERVE

120g wild rice

1. First make the peanut sauce. Heat the olive oil in a frying pan and fry the peanuts, garlic, chilli and turmeric together until very aromatic (about 5 minutes). Remove from the oil with a slotted spoon and put into a pestle and mortar – or a blender, if you're feeling lazy!

2. Grind the peanut mix with the soy sauce and lime juice. Add the water, little by little, until the desired consistency is reached. Set aside half of the peanut sauce for lunch tomorrow, in a covered container in the fridge.

3. Cook the rice according to the packet instructions.

4. To make the kebabs, thread all the vegetables and tempeh onto the skewers. Heat the grill (or a griddle pan if you don't have a grill) and cook on a medium–high heat for 8–10 minutes, turning every now and then, until the vegetables are soft and cooked all over.

5. Serve the rice in a bowl piled with the kebabs and the peanut sauce drizzled over.

BREAKFAST

Layered summer fruit parfait with coconut yoghurt and granola

Under 650 calories

The layers in this fruit parfait are really pretty. We eat with our eyes, so having pretty food really is important – and this recipe really is photogenic.

100g raspberries

100g strawberries, chopped into pieces

100g coconut yoghurt (from last week's shopping list!)

60g quinoa granola with dried raspberries and cacao nibs (from Saturday Week 2 breakfast)

4 tbsp chia jam (from Saturday Week 1 breakfast)

50g dessicated coconut

---

1. In two tall glasses, layer the fruit, coconut yoghurt and granola.

2. Top with the chia jam and desiccated coconut to serve.

LUNCH

Sourdough fattoush with butter beans

Under 500 calories

Fattoush is a traditional Levantine bread salad which is made from mixed green or other vegetables and toasted or fried pieces of (traditionally) flatbread. Using sourdough gives this salad a different twist, and the addition of butter beans adds extra protein.

If you're preparing this ahead of time and taking it to work, keep the dressing separate and add it when you are ready to eat, so the bread doesn't go soggy. You will not use all the salad dressing here, so you can keep the rest in the fridge for later use. It keeps well for at least one week – and will be needed for Thursday's lunch!

FOR THE SALAD

2 slices of sourdough
200g cherry tomatoes, halved
¼ cucumber, thinly sliced
2 spring onions, thinly sliced
1 little gem lettuce, cut into
    thin strips
1 large bunch of flat-leaf
    parsley, finely chopped
1 large bunch of mint

FOR THE DRESSING

Juice of 1 lemon
30ml pomegranate molasses
1 garlic clove, minced
30ml white wine vinegar
100ml olive oil

---

1. To make the dressing, put all the ingredients except the olive oil into a bowl and whisk until well combined. Add the olive oil, a small amount at a time, whisking thoroughly until fully incorporated.

2. Toast the sourdough.

3. To make the salad, combine all the remaining ingredients in a serving bowl, then tear the sourdough toast over the top roughly. Pour over the dressing evenly and serve immediately.

DINNER

Sweet potato and chickpea curry with a spiced tomato salad

Under 600 calories

This curry couldn't be easier to make – everything goes into one pot! The lemongrass, mustard seeds and cardamom make the curry lovely and aromatic, rather than particularly spicy. If you love 'hot' food you can always add extra chilli flakes. I personally like to eat my curry with some pan-fried kale, too, but you can serve it with rice (brown or basmati rice are lower-GI options) or naan bread (although this is about 400 calories a slice!).

FOR THE CURRY
1 sweet potato, peeled and cut
    into 2cm cubes
2 tsp olive oil
1 tsp chilli flakes
Juice of 1 lime
½ white onion, diced
3 tsp red Thai curry paste
2 lemongrass sticks, bashed
1 tsp mustard seeds
6 cardamom pods
1 tsp turmeric
1 x 400ml tin reduced-fat
    coconut milk

1 x 400g tin chickpeas, drained
    and rinsed

FOR THE SALAD
1 tsp cumin seeds
400g cherry tomatoes, halved
1 small cucumber, diced
1 red onion, diced
Small handful of coriander,
    finely chopped
Juice of 1 lime
2 tbsp olive oil

1. Preheat the oven to 180°C/160°C fan/350°F/gas mark 4.

2. Pop the sweet potato into a baking tray and coat the cubes in 1 teaspoon of olive oil, chilli flakes and lime juice, then roast them in the oven for about 25 minutes, until they are tender when pierced with a knife.

3. Meanwhile, in a saucepan, heat 1 teaspoon of olive oil. When the oil is sizzling hot, add the onion and fry for a few minutes until softened and translucent.

4. Add all the spices to the saucepan (red Thai curry paste, lemongrass sticks, mustard seeds, cardamom pods and turmeric) and continue to fry until the mixture is fragrant.

5. When the sweet potato is tender, add it to the pan along with the coconut milk and chickpeas. Cook for 5 minutes to make sure the curry is heated right through, then pick out the lemongrass and cardamom pods.

6. Meanwhile, make the salad. Dry-fry the cumin seeds in a frying pan for a few minutes, until aromatic, shaking the pan to make sure they don't burn. Toss all the remaining ingredients except the lime juice and olive oil in a bowl to combine. Tip half of the tomato salad into a sealable container for lunch tomorrow and store in the fridge – put the lime juice and olive oil into a little pot ready to dress the salad just before eating.

7. Add the lime juice and olive oil to the salad and mix so that the vegetables are well coated in the dressing. Serve the dressed salad with the curry.

BREAKFAST

Cacao, date and banana smoothie

Under 550 calories

This is a sweet, chocolatey smoothie. It is very filling, and great for breakfast but also as a snack. If you prefer it really cold, serve it over ice.

600ml hazelnut milk

2 bananas, broken into chunks

1 avocado, halved, stoned and peeled

2 scoops of soya protein powder (or other vegan alternative, if preferred)

4 tbsp cacao powder

---

1. Combine all the ingredients in a blender and blitz until smooth and thoroughly mixed.

2. Divide the smoothie among two glasses.

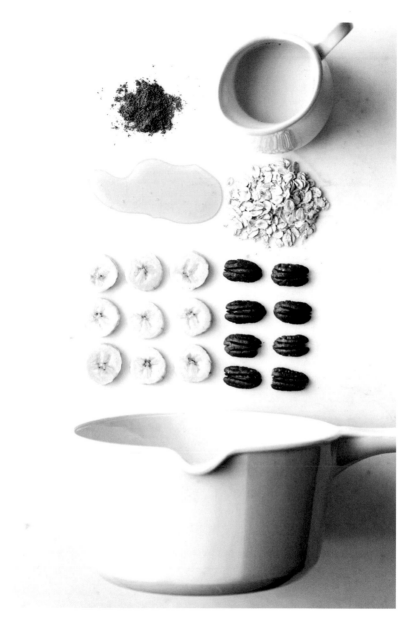

Week 1 – Friday – Breakfast
Banana, maple syrup and pecan porridge

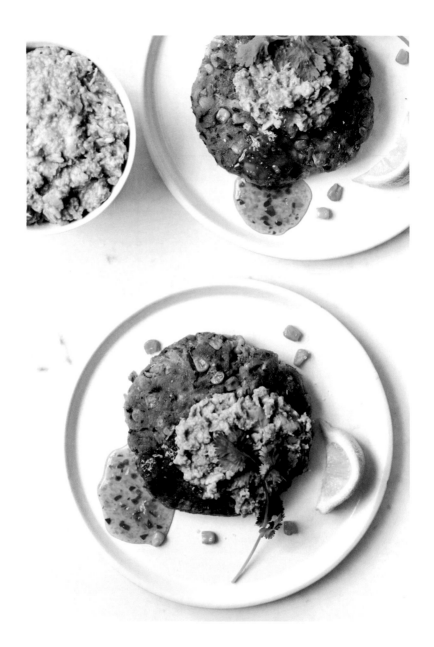

Week 4 – Sunday – Breakfast
Spicy sweetcorn fritters with avocado and coriander

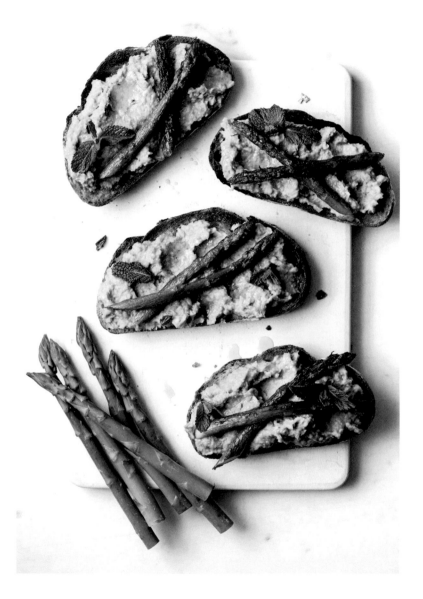

Week 2 – Saturday – Lunch
Broad bean, asparagus and mint tartine

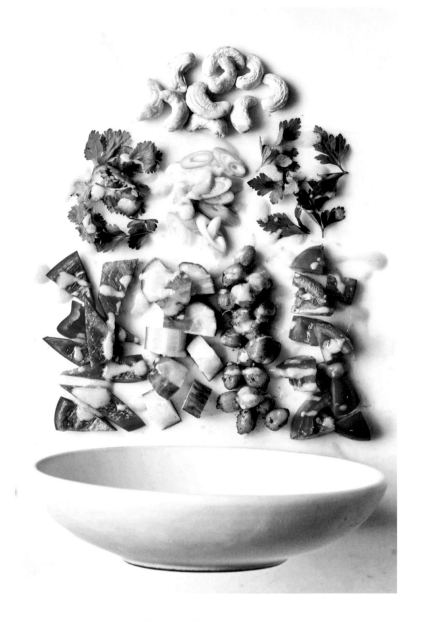

Week 4 – Sunday– Lunch
Toasted spiced chickpea salad

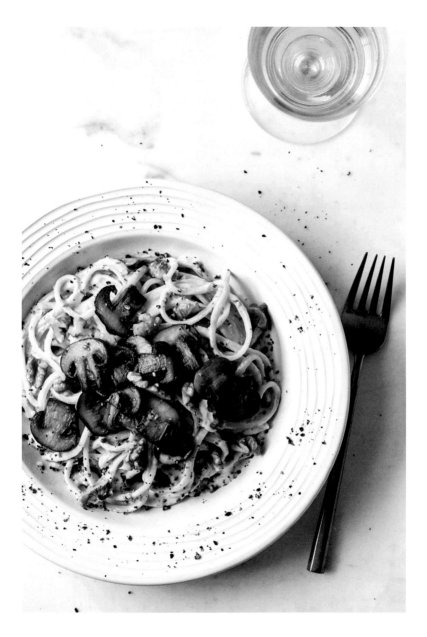

Week 1 – Friday – Dinner
Linguine with a mushroom and chestnut sauce

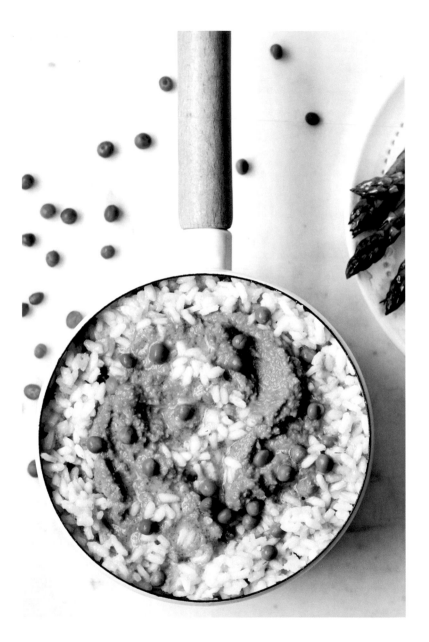

Week 2 – Friday – Dinner
Lemon and pea risotto with roasted asparagus spears

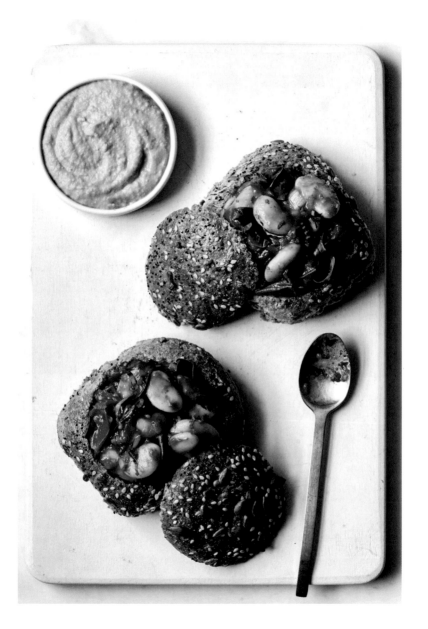

Week 4 – Friday – Dinner
'Beany' chow

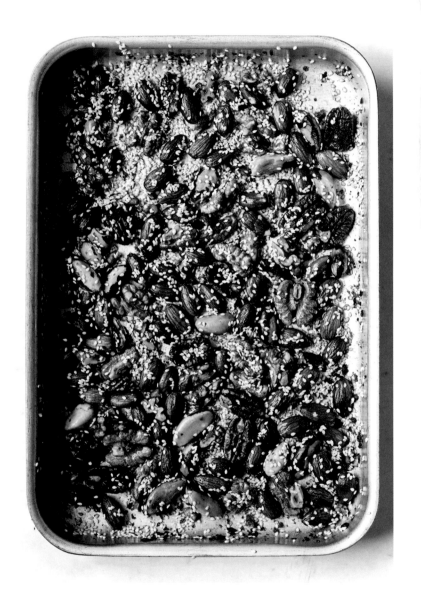

Snack
Sweet sesame roasted nuts

LUNCH

Indian-spiced tomato and white bean salad

Under 400 calories

By using the leftover tomato salad from Monday's dinner, this lunch could not be easier to prepare. If you really want to cheat, you can get couscous that is already cooked, then all you need to do is toss the ingredients together.

Tomato salad (from Monday's dinner)	drained and rinsed
75g couscous	Handful of mint, chopped
1 x 400g tin butter beans,	Handful of coriander, chopped

1. Prepare the couscous according to the packet instructions.

2. Mix the couscous thoroughly with the tomato salad, butter beans and herbs in a large serving bowl and serve immediately.

DINNER

Quinoa bowl – harissa-roasted aubergine, garlic mushrooms, spinach and hummus

Under 700 calories

This quinoa bowl is a classic flavour combination. The hummus is essential here as it adds a creamy texture which is great with the vegetables but also provides essential protein.

While the aubergine is roasting, take a look at the recipes for breakfast and lunch tomorrow, as you need to prepare these in advance.

FOR THE QUINOA BOWL	FOR THE HUMMUS
1 aubergine, cut into small chunks	1 x 400g tin chickpeas, drained and rinsed
1 tbsp harissa paste	2 tbsp olive oil
2 tbsp olive oil	1 garlic clove
1 tsp chilli flakes	Juice of 1 lemon
120g quinoa	2 tbsp harissa paste
150g chestnut mushrooms	1 tbsp tomato purée
2 garlic cloves, crushed	½ tsp paprika, to garnish
200g spinach	

Get ahead

If you have time, steps 1–4 of tomorrow's lunch (the Gado-gado with quinoa) are best done the night before, for lunch, but it's not essential.

1. Preheat the oven to 180°C/160°C fan/350°F/gas mark 4.

2. Place the aubergine chunks in a roasting tin with the harissa, 1 tablespoon of the olive oil and the chilli flakes, and roast for 30 minutes.

3. While the aubergine is roasting, make the hummus. Blend all the ingredients together, except the paprika, until smooth. Set aside half for dinner on Thursday and spoon the rest into a bowl and sprinkle with the paprika.

4. Cook the quinoa according to the packet instructions.

5. To make the garlicky mushrooms, sauté the mushrooms and garlic in the remaining olive oil in a dry frying pan for about 5 minutes, until they begin to go brown on the outside and slightly crispy. Undercooked mushrooms are soggy – so cook them for a little longer if in doubt.

6. Set the mushrooms aside in a bowl and use the same frying pan to cook the spinach over a medium heat. If you use a non-stick pan, you shouldn't need any more oil, but if not, add a little extra so the spinach doesn't stick. Stir the spinach until it wilts.

7. Assemble the quinoa bowl, starting with the quinoa on the bottom and layer up with the aubergine, mushrooms and spinach. Top with the hummus.

BREAKFAST

Apple and ginger bircher muesli

Under 550 calories

The sweetness from the apple and the tanginess from the ginger makes this breakfast a real winner. You can even experiment with your own flavours of bircher muesli – just make sure you keep the ratio of oats to liquid the same and add any fruits, nuts and seeds that you like.

80g rolled oats

400ml hazelnut milk

2 tbsp maple syrup

1 tsp vanilla extract

1 thumb-sized piece of root
    ginger, finely grated

50g linseeds

1 tsp ground cinnamon

2 dessert apples, coarsely
    grated

30g dried cranberries

30g sultanas

---

1. Combine the oats, hazelnut milk, maple syrup, vanilla extract, ginger, linseeds and cinnamon in a large bowl, cover and leave in the fridge overnight.

2. In the morning, stir through the apple and divide among two bowls.

3. Serve topped with the cranberries and sultanas.

LUNCH

Gado-gado with quinoa

Under 750 calories

This is a traditional Balinese salad made with tempeh and tofu. Here you'll use tempeh, although firm tofu is OK if you struggle to find tempeh. The quinoa is a new addition to provide slow-release carbohydrate to keep you going through the afternoon.

---

2 tbsp olive oil
300g tempeh, cut into 2cm
   chunks
100g quinoa
100g green beans

½ cucumber, cut into small
   chunks
Peanut sauce (leftover from
   Sunday's dinner)

---

1. Heat the olive oil in a pan over a high heat, then add the tempeh and stir-fry until really crispy on the outside.

2. Cook the quinoa according to the packet instructions.

3. Steam the green beans over a pan of simmering water for about 5 minutes, then drain. Immediately pour cold water over them, so they stop cooking and retain their lovely green colour. Leave all the ingredients to cool.

4. To assemble the salad, simply mix all tempeh, vegetables and quinoa together, and dress with the peanut sauce.

DINNER

Vegan quinoa sushi

Under 500 calories excluding extras

Sushi is a brilliant food to make with friends. Once you have cooked the rice and prepared the vegetables to go inside, you can sit down and roll this with friends. It actually makes a great dinner party meal. Adding quinoa gives this dish extra protein, which is important when you are removing the traditional protein source of raw fish for a vegan diet.

150g quinoa
½ tbsp rice wine vinegar
1 tsp sugar
¼ tsp salt
3 sheets of sushi nori
1 avocado, thinly sliced
1 carrot, peeled and thinly sliced
¼ cucumber, thinly sliced

EXTRAS TO SERVE (OPTIONAL)
Soy sauce
Pickled ginger
Wasabi paste

1. Cook the quinoa according to the packet instructions and allow to cool.

2. Mix the rice wine vinegar, sugar and salt together, then pour over the quinoa.

3. Lay the sushi nori sheets shiny side down. Divide the quinoa between the sheets, spreading it out in an even layer over the nearest half of the nori sheet, then add the vegetables in a line down the middle of the quinoa.

4. Roll tightly and ensure the nori sticks to itself to seal the sushi roll.

5. Using a very sharp knife, slice the nori 'sausage' into coins about 4cm thick and place them on a plate.

6. Serve with soy sauce, pickled ginger and wasabi paste, if you like.

BREAKFAST

Tropical popical smoothie

Under 500 calories

This smoothie makes you feel like you're on holiday! The orange juice is tangy with a smooth and creamy twist from the coconut milk – it really is delicious.

---

2 bananas
130g fresh pineapple chunks
400ml orange juice
200ml coconut milk (keep the rest of the tin in a sealed

Tupperware in the fridge for next Monday's dinner)
Handful of ice cubes
40g bran flakes

---

1. Put all the ingredients into a blender and blitz together until smooth.

2. Divide the smoothie among two glasses and serve.

LUNCH

Mango, tomato and basil salad

Under 600 calories

This salad is really fresh; the flavours of mango, tomato and basil are quite strong and work really well together, and the pine nuts provide added crunch!

120g quinoa	2 plum tomatoes
70g pine nuts	Rocket leaves
1 small mango, cut into small chunks	Small bunch of basil, chopped
	1 avocado, cut into cubes

1. Cook the quinoa according to the packet instructions.

2. Toast the pine nuts in a shallow frying pan until aromatic, for about 3 minutes, shaking the pan to prevent them from burning.

3. Mix all the ingredients together, then divide among two bowls to serve.

DINNER

Spinach crepes with a pepper filling

Under 600 calories

Pancakes do not need to be saved for breakfasts only – savoury crepes are delicious. The addition of spinach to the batter makes the mixture hold together really well and gives the crepes a lovely crunch, while also making them visually beautiful and a lovely green colour.

FOR THE PANCAKES
1 tbsp linseeds
3 tbsp water
100g spinach
Small bunch of flat-leaf parsley
60g plain flour
120ml almond milk
Zest of 1 lemon
Salt and pepper, to taste
1 tsp olive oil

ROASTED PEPPER FILLING
2 red peppers
1 garlic clove, chopped
1 tbsp olive oil

TO SERVE
Hummus (from Tuesday's
    dinner)
Small bunch of flat-leaf
    parsley, chopped

1. Preheat the oven to 180°C/160°C fan/350°F/gas mark 4.

2. Mix the linseeds and water in a cup and leave to stand for half an hour, until they form a 'jelly'.

3. Meanwhile, prepare the roasted peppers. Cut them into strips and place on a baking tray with the garlic, then drizzle with the olive oil. Using your hands, toss the peppers so they are well coated in the garlic and olive oil, and roast for 25 minutes.

4. In a food processor, blend the spinach and parsley to a paste.

5. Add the linseed 'jelly', flour, almond milk, lemon zest, salt and pepper to the blender, and pulse until smooth.

6. Heat the olive oil in a shallow, non-stick frying pan.

7. Pour about three-quarters of a cup of the mixture into the frying pan, tilting the pan so that the pancake batter spreads quickly across the base. When you can see the edges of the batter beginning to lighten in colour, the pancake is about done on one side. Flip it over and cook on the other side.

8. Serve the pancakes stuffed with the peppers, hummus and extra parsley.

BREAKFAST

Porridge with vanilla poached plums

Under 500 calories

Poaching is a great way to soften fruit, so don't worry if you can't find perfectly ripe plums. You can also try this with other stone fruit, such as apricots or nectarines.

50g dark muscovado sugar	6 plums, halved, stones
50ml water	removed
2 tsp vanilla extract	120g rolled oats
	400ml almond milk

1. First make the poached plums. In a saucepan over a medium heat, dissolve the sugar in the water. Add the vanilla extract and plums and simmer for 10 minutes until the plums have softened.

2. While the plums cook, make the porridge. Put the oats and nut milk into a saucepan over a low heat. Stir continuously for 5–10 minutes, until all the liquid is absorbed.

3. Divide the porridge among two bowls and serve topped with the plums.

LUNCH

Turkish tomato salad with coconut haydari

Under 450 calories without pitta, under 600 calories with pitta

Haydari is a Turkish dish of herbs and spices, combined with garlic and yoghurt. Using coconut yoghurt gives this dish a slightly different flavour, which works really well with the tomatoes and peppers. If you want, you can serve with warm pittas on the side.

FOR THE SALAD

2 plum tomatoes, diced

2 Romano peppers, deseeded and diced

1 tsp chilli flakes

1 red onion, diced

1 tsp harissa paste

2 spring onions, finely sliced

1 tbsp olive oil

1 tbsp pomegranate molasses

1 tsp white wine vinegar

200g ready-to-eat quinoa and lentil mix

Salt and pepper, to taste

FOR THE COCONUT HAYDARI

Coconut yoghurt (leftover from last week)

Small bunch of flat-leaf parsley, chopped

Small bunch of mint, chopped

---

1. Mix together all the salad ingredients.

2. To make the coconut haydari, mix all the ingredients together until well combined.

3. Top the salad with the coconut haydari.

DINNER

Quinoa-stuffed peppers with Moroccan flavours

Under 550 calories

The capers, preserved lemon and basil mean that these peppers are not only stuffed with quinoa, they are filled with flavour. This recipe also demonstrates how to make breadcrumbs, which is something you can do for many recipes throughout the book, too.

2 Romano peppers, sliced in half lengthways
1 slice of sourdough toast
110g quinoa
¼ preserved lemon, diced
Juice of 1 lemon
2 spring onions, sliced thinly
1 garlic clove, diced

Handful of basil, roughly chopped
3 tbsp capers, drained and rinsed
50g flaked almonds
Pepper, to taste
2 tsp olive oil

1. Preheat the oven to 200°C/180°C fan/400°F/gas mark 6.

2. Pop the peppers into a separate roasting tin, cut side up, and roast them for 12 minutes until fairly soft. Leave the oven on.

3. Meanwhile, pulse the sourdough toast in a blender until fine crumbs form, then scatter them in a roasting tin and cook in the oven for about 10 minutes to dry out. Cook the quinoa according to the packet instructions.

4. When the quinoa is cooked, add all the remaining ingredients to the pan and fork through until well combined. Use this quinoa mix to stuff the peppers.

5. Sprinkle the top of the stuffed peppers with the toasted breadcrumbs and olive oil.

6. Bake for about 10 minutes, until the quinoa and breadcrumbs are crunchy on top.

Recipes: Week 4

N.B. Each meal serves two people
unless otherwise stated.

SHOPPING LIST

Dairy alternatives

- [ ] 2 litres soya milk
- [ ] 1 litre hazelnut milk
- [ ] 1 litre almond milk
- [ ] 1 x 255g tub 'Free From' soft cheese

Fruit and vegetables

- [ ] 2 white onions
- [ ] 2 red onions
- [ ] 1 potato (large)
- [ ] 2 sweet potatoes (1 large)
- [ ] 6 spring onions
- [ ] 1 avocado
- [ ] 12 cherry tomoatoes
- [ ] 250g baby spinach
- [ ] 2 red peppers
- [ ] 1 bag rocket
- [ ] 18 plum tomatoes
- [ ] 1 small cucumber
- [ ] 150g green beans
- [ ] 1 celeriac
- [ ] 3 carrots

- [ ] 220g chestnut mushrooms
- [ ] 200g wild mushrooms
- [ ] 3 courgettes
- [ ] 300g sundried tomatoes
- [ ] 1 x 280g jar of artichoke hearts
- [ ] 2 limes
- [ ] 5 lemons
- [ ] 350g frozen strawberries
- [ ] 2 pears
- [ ] 8 bananas (put two in the freezer!)
- [ ] 50g pomegranate seeds
- [ ] 1 x 410g tin pears

Carbohydrate staples

- [ ] 1 pizza base
- [ ] 4 crusty wholemeal rolls
- [ ] 2 vegan naan breads (or flatbreads if you can't find vegan naans)

Dried store foods

☐ 1 x 400g tin sweetcorn

☐ 1 x 198g tin sweetcorn

☐ 200ml coconut milk
(leftover from last week)

☐ 100g ground almonds

☐ 100g silken tofu

☐ 2 x 400g tins chickpeas

☐ 1 x 400g tin red kidney
beans

☐ 1 x 400g tin butter beans

☐ Dried black lentils

☐ 1 x 227g tin chopped
tomatoes

☐ 100ml coconut cream

☐ 250g ready-cooked puy
lentils

Other

☐ Almond butter

☐ 4–6 vegan sausages

☐ 130g pine nuts (leftover
from week 2)

☐ 100g cashews

☐ Tamarind paste

☐ 70g coconut flakes

Fresh herbs

☐ Coriander*

☐ Parsley*

*You may not need to buy
these if you have leftovers
from previous weeks.

MENU

	Breakfast	Lunch	Dinner
Saturday	Banana, fig and pear muffins	Raw carrot gazpacho	Vegan sausages with truffle mash
Sunday	Spicy sweetcorn fritters with avocado and coriander	Toasted spiced chickpea salad	Vegan pizzas with roasted tomato hummus
Monday	Strawberry and soya breakfast smoothie	Sweetcorn and bean wrap	Coconut and tamarind curry
Tuesday	Pear and date bircher muesli	Hummus and grilled courgette wrap	Mushroom and rocket polenta tart with gremolata
Wednesday	Almond butter, pomegranate and fig	Lentil salad with gremolata	Spaghetti with a creamy artichoke sauce

	Breakfast	Lunch	Dinner
Thursday	Berry and vanilla chia pudding with a crunchy granola topping	Tartine with artichoke paté and pan-fried vegetables	Coconut and tomato daal with a zesty mango salad
Friday	Peanut butter and frozen banana smoothie	Quinoa mango salad	'Beany' chow

BREAKFAST

Banana, fig and pear muffins

Under 300 calories per muffin

This recipe makes 12 muffins – you can freeze any leftovers for breakfasts or snacks on another day. Just get them out of the freezer the night before and take them out for an on-the-go breakfast or mid-morning nibble. A serving is two muffins.

90g rolled oats	1 x 400g tin pears in natural
100g ground almonds	juice, chopped
80g linseeds	2 tsp ground cinnamon
4 bananas	30ml maple syrup
120ml water	100g dried figs, chopped

1. Preheat the oven to 180°C/160°C fan/350°F/gas mark 4. Line a 12-hole muffin tin with muffin cases.

2. In a blender, blitz the oats, almonds and linseeds to a smooth powder.

3. Add the bananas, water, juice from the tinned pears, cinnamon and maple syrup and blend again until smooth.

4. Transfer the batter to a large mixing bowl.

5. Stir the chopped figs and pears into the batter. Divide the batter carefully among the 12 muffin cases.

6. Bake in the oven for 30–40 minutes. When they are done, you should be able to insert a knife into the centre and it will come out clean.

7. Allow to cool in the tin, then transfer to a wire rack to cool completely before eating or storing.

LUNCH

Raw carrot gazpacho

Under 500 calories including buttered roll

Gazpacho is an Andalusian soup made of raw blended vegetables and is served cold. This one is made of carrots, so it is a beautiful vibrant orange.

FOR THE SOUP
2 large carrots, washed and
    roughly chopped, skin on
Large bunch of coriander
50g cashews
240ml almond milk
Juice of ½ lime

A thumb-sized knob of root
    ginger, grated
¼ tsp chilli flakes
Salt and pepper, to taste

TO SERVE
2 crusty wholemeal rolls
Vegan butter

1. To make the soup, combine all the ingredients in a blender and blitz until smooth. You may want to add some water, depending on how thick you like your soup.

2. Push the soup through a sieve, so it is really smooth, into a bowl.

3. Warm the bread rolls through and serve spread with vegan butter alongside the soup.

DINNER

Vegan sausages with truffle mash

Under 600 calories

Vegan sausages are available from most supermarkets, often in the frozen section. There are many different brands, so when choosing, make sure you look at the ingredients list. Some people worry that processed foods (such as vegan sausages) are really bad for you and should be avoided, but that's not necessarily the case. It's about moderation; it's OK to eat some processed foods, as they can make your diet more practical, but it is always worth checking the sugar and salt content.

4–6 vegan sausages
(depending on the size)

1 tsp olive oil

2 garlic cloves, chopped

150g green beans

FOR THE MASH

1 large potato, tough outside

skin removed, flesh chopped
into small chunks

2 tbsp truffle-infused olive oil

1 tsp vegan butter

Ground nutmeg (optional),
to taste

Knob of vegan butter

Salt and pepper, to taste

---

1. Cook the sausages according to the packet instructions.

2. Meanwhile, boil the potato in a pan of salted water for about 10 minutes. Drain and return to the saucepan, then put back on the heat for about 1 minute. All the extra moisture will evaporate, preventing your mash going 'soggy'.

3. Mash the potato thoroughly, adding the olive oil, vegan butter, salt, pepper and nutmeg (if using). Set aside.

4. In a small saucepan, heat the olive oil and fry the garlic.

5. Boil the green beans for about 4 minutes, drain, then pour over the hot oil and garlic.

6. Serve the mash piled high with the sausages and green beans.

Get ahead

Freeze two of the bananas from your shopping basket for Friday's breakfast, if you haven't already done so.

BREAKFAST

Spicy sweetcorn fritters with avocado and coriander

Under 650 calories

Unlike many fritter recipes, this batter holds together really well so these are so easy to cook. When topped with avocado and herbs, they look very pretty, too. This dish is served with sweet chilli sauce, which is high in sugar, so only use a little for flavour.

FOR THE FRITTERS
1 large sweet potato, cut into
   chunks
1 red onion, cut into chunks
2 garlic cloves, cut into chunks
1½ tbsp olive oil
Salt, pepper, chilli flakes, to
   taste
50ml water
1 x 400g tin sweetcorn
Small bunch of coriander, finely
   chopped

2 spring onions, finely sliced
50g plain flour, plus extra for
   dusting
1 avocado

TO SERVE
Juice of 1 lemon
Low-sugar sweet chilli sauce
Small bunch of coriander, finely
   chopped

1. Preheat the oven to 180°C/160°C fan/350°F/gas mark 4.

2. Put the sweet potato, red onion and garlic into a roasting dish, drizzle with ½ a tablespoon of olive oil, and sprinkle with the salt, pepper and chilli flakes. Roast the vegetables in the oven for 30 minutes, until soft.

3. When the vegetables are cooked through, put them into a blender with the water and blitz until fairly smooth. Scoop out into a mixing bowl.

4. Add the sweetcorn, coriander, spring onions and flour to the mixing bowl and combine thoroughly with the roast vegetable purée.

5. On a floured surface, shape the mixture into two patties. If the mixture is too wet, you can add some more flour. If it is a bit dry, you can add more water. You want the patties to hold together.

6. In a shallow frying pan, heat the remaining olive oil and fry the patties for about 5 minutes on each side, until browned and slightly crispy.

7. Meanwhile, scoop out the avocado flesh and mash roughly in a bowl with the lemon juice.

8. Serve the hot fritters topped with avocado, sweet chilli sauce and coriander.

LUNCH

Toasted spiced chickpea salad

Under 600 calories

The spiced chickpeas are delicious in this salad, as they give a warming flavour and a nice little crunch. You can always make extra for snacks, too, as they'll keep well for up to one week in an airtight container.

FOR THE CHICKPEA SALAD
1 x 400g tin chickpeas, drained and rinsed
1 tbsp olive oil
4 cardamom pods, ground in a pestle and mortar
1½ tsp ground allspice
1 tsp ground cumin
1 small cucumber, diced
2 large tomatoes, diced
1 red pepper, deseeded and diced
Small bunch of coriander, chopped
Small bunch of flat-leaf parsley, chopped
50g cashews
2 spring onions, finely sliced

FOR THE DRESSING
Zest and juice of 1 lemon
1 tbsp tahini
2 tbsp olive oil
1 garlic clove, minced
1 tsp balsamic vinegar

1. Preheat the oven to 180°C/160°C fan/350°F/gas mark 4.

2. Toss the chickpeas in the oil and spices, then bake for 15 minutes until crispy.

3. Meanwhile, make the dressing by combining all the ingredients in a bowl.

4. Toss the chickpeas with all the salad vegetables in a large serving bowl and drizzle the salad dressing on top.

DINNER

Vegan pizza with roasted tomato hummus

Under 750 calories

This vegan pizza is topped with hummus instead of cheese. Vegan cheeses are available, but lots of people don't like them, so hummus is a great alternative.

FOR THE PIZZA
1 pizza base
2 tbsp tomato purée
1 red pepper, deseeded and
   sliced
1 x 400g tin sweetcorn,
   drained and half saved for
   tomorrow's lunch
4 tsp dried oregano
Handful of rocket leaves,
   to serve

FOR THE ROASTED
TOMATOES
10 plum tomatoes, halved
1 tbsp olive oil

1 tbsp balsamic vinegar
2 tsp dried oregano
Salt and pepper, to taste

FOR THE HUMMUS
1 x 400g tin chickpeas,
   drained and rinsed
2 tbsp olive oil
Juice of 1 lemon
2 tsp tahini
1 tsp paprika
1 tsp ground cumin
3 tbsp water

1. Preheat the oven to 220°C/200°C fan/425°F/gas mark 7.

2. Start by making the roasted tomatoes. In a baking tray, lay the tomatoes cut-side up, drizzle all over with the oil and balsamic vinegar and scatter over the oregano and salt and pepper. Roast for about 20 minutes, until soft. Leave the oven on.

3. To make the hummus, put the chickpeas, olive oil, lemon juice, tahini, paprika and cumin in a blender and blitz together until completely smooth. Then take half of the roasted tomatoes and blend them into the mix. Add the water, a small amount at a time, until you reach the desired consistency.

4. Cover the pizza base with tomato purée, then top with the red pepper, sweetcorn, dried oregano and the remaining roasted tomatoes. Dollop 6 teaspoons of hummus onto the pizza and keep the leftover hummus in a covered bowl in the fridge – you will need this for three other meals in the week. Bake the pizza for about 15 minutes, until the base is crispy and the hummus is soft and hot. Serve topped with rocket.

BREAKFAST

Strawberry and soya breakfast smoothie

Under 350 calories

The addition of soya to this smoothie adds some important extra protein and makes it taste delicious. Make sure you buy silken tofu as it has a lovely creamy consistency; it is normally available in the Asian foods aisle of the supermarket.

100g silken tofu	40g bran flakes
600ml soya milk	240g frozen strawberries

1. Put all the ingredients in a blender and blitz together until smooth.

2. Add some ice cubes to two glasses, pour in the smoothie and serve.

LUNCH

Sweetcorn and bean wrap

Under 500 calories

This lunch is really filling, thanks to the red kidney beans. It can be prepared in minutes, making it the perfect lunch to take to work, just roll and wrap for later!

---

2 flour tortilla wraps
4 tbsp tomato hummus (from
    Sunday's dinner)
1 x 200g tin sweetcorn
    (leftover from last night's
    dinner)

1 x 400g tin red kidney beans,
    drained and rinsed
2 large handfuls of rocket
    leaves

---

1. Heat the tortillas according to the packet instructions, then spread them with hummus.

2. Divide the sweetcorn, beans and rocket among the wraps, then roll up and serve.

DINNER

Tamarind and coconut curry with quinoa

Under 750 calories

This curry is extremely easy to make, but full of flavour. The crunchy coconut flakes and coriander leaves scattered on top add a lovely texture to the dish. Here the curry is served with quinoa, as a good protein source, but you can use rice if you prefer.

1 tbsp olive oil
1 red onion, peeled and diced
1 tsp chilli flakes
2 garlic cloves, finely chopped
Thumb-sized piece of root
    ginger, peeled and finely
    chopped
1 small bunch of coriander,
    leaves and stalks chopped

    separately
1 tsp mustard seeds
1 sweet potato
1 x 200ml tin coconut milk
1 x 227g tin tomatoes
1 tbsp tamarind paste
120g quinoa
70g coconut flakes

1. Put the olive oil, red onion, chilli, garlic and ginger into a large saucepan over a medium heat and cook for about 5 minutes, until the onion is browned and very aromatic. Add the coriander stalks, fennel seeds and mustard seeds and cook for a further 3 minutes until the mustard seeds begin to pop.

2. Add the sweet potato, coconut milk, tomatoes and tamarind paste and simmer for about 20 minutes until the sauce has thickened and the sweet potato is soft.

3. While the curry is simmering, cook the quinoa according to the packet instructions.

4. Toast the coconut flakes in a dry frying pan over a medium heat for about 5 minutes, stirring regularly. They will begin to turn a golden brown colour and become very aromatic, at which point, remove them from the heat. Be careful they don't burn.

5. Serve the curry, sprinkled with the toasted coconut flakes and the coriander leaves.

Get ahead

Tonight you need to start preparing the bircher muesli for tomorrow's breakfast.

BREAKFAST

Pear and date bircher muesli

Under 700 calories

This bircher muesli is mostly made the night before so it is a really quick, on-the-go breakfast. The addition of the toasted pistachios gives it a little extra crunch!

80g rolled oats
300ml soya milk
2 tbsp maple syrup
20g linseeds
1 tsp vanilla extract

50g pistachio nuts
2 pears, peeled, cored and
   sliced
50g medjool dates

---

1. Combine the oats, milk, maple syrup, linseeds and vanilla extract in a large bowl and put in the fridge, covered, overnight.

2. In the morning, toast the pistachios in a dry frying pan for about 3 minutes, until fragrant, shaking the pan occasionally to prevent them from burning.

3. Top the bircher muesli with the nuts, pears and dates.

LUNCH

Hummus and grilled courgette wrap

Under 600 calories

This lunch uses grilled courgettes. However, if you are not able to cook during the day, for example you are at work without the facilities, raw courgettes are delicious, too.

2 courgettes, medium, cut lengthways into 'batons'	dinner)
2 tsp olive oil	2 large handfuls of rocket leaves
2 flour tortilla wraps	75g sundried tomatoes
2 tbsp tomato hummus (leftover from Sunday's	50g pine nuts
	Salt and pepper, to taste

1. Brush both sides of the courgette slices with the oil and sprinkle with the salt and pepper.

2. On a griddle pan (or in a frying pan), grill the courgettes until tender and slightly browned, for about 4 minutes each side.

3. Lay out the wraps and spread with hummus, then pile up the rocket and sundried tomatoes, scattering with the pine nuts. Fold the wrap to seal and serve.

DINNER

Mushroom and rocket polenta tart with gremolata

Under 600 calories

This tart is really pretty – and so easy to make. The earthy mushrooms taste amazing with the 'zing' from the gremolata. You'll have much more gremolata than you need, so put the rest in a sterilised jar (see page 46) in the fridge for lunch tomorrow and for other meals.

FOR THE GREMOLATA
1 garlic clove, chopped
Zest and juice of 1 lemon
Small bunch of flat-leaf
    parsley, chopped finely

FOR THE POLENTA
400ml soya milk
1 tsp black peppercorns
2 sprigs of rosemary
1 bay leaf
100g polenta

1 tbsp truffle-infused olive oil
2 large handfuls of rocket
    leaves

FOR THE MUSHROOMS
2 tbsp olive oil
1 white onion, diced
4 garlic cloves, crushed
220g chestnut mushrooms
200g wild mushrooms
Salt and pepper, to taste

1. First, make the gremolata by combining all the ingredients in a small bowl.

2. Start on the polenta. On the hob, heat the soya milk in a saucepan with the peppercorns, rosemary and bay leaf. Heat until almost boiling, then take off the heat and allow to cool. The further in advance you can do this the better, to allow the herbs to infuse the soya milk.

3. Strain the milk to remove the herbs and peppercorns. Add the polenta, a small amount at a time, to the herby soya milk and whisk over a medium heat, until all the moisture is absorbed and the polenta is cooked through. You may need some extra liquid (such as boiling water from the kettle) depending on the cooking instructions on the packet, as all polenta differs. Preheat the oven to 180°C/160°C fan/350°F/gas mark 4.

4. For the mushrooms, heat the olive oil in an ovenproof frying pan, then add the onion and garlic and sauté for about 3 minutes, until slightly soft. Add the mushrooms and sauté for another 7 minutes, until golden brown.

5. Remove the polenta from the heat, add the truffle oil and rocket and stir thoroughly to mix.

6. Pour the polenta over the mushrooms and put the pan in the oven for 20 minutes.

7. Serve the dish hot, drizzled with the gremolata.

BREAKFAST

Almond butter and fig porridge

Under 550 calories

Porridge is a great way to start the day, because it is really high in slow release carbohydrates to fuel you through the morning. Cooking with bananas in the porridge will make it deliciously sweet, as the bananas release some of their natural sugars.

80g rolled oats	½ tsp mixed spice
320ml almond milk	150g figs, roughly chopped
2 medium bananas, cut into coins	2 tsp almond butter
	50g pomegranate seeds

1. Put the oats, nut milk, bananas and mixed spice into a saucepan over a low heat and stir continuously for 5–10 minutes, until all the liquid is absorbed and the bananas are very soft.

2. Divide the porridge among two bowls and top with the chopped figs, some almond butter and the pomegranate seeds.

LUNCH

Lentil salad with gremolata

Under 300 calories

This lunch is really filling thanks to the lentils. Often people can find lentils bland, but with the punchy gremolata this salad is far from boring. The addition of spinach leaves gives a nice little crunch, and the tomatoes make it colourful.

250g ready-cooked puy lentils
2 tomatoes, diced
200g baby spinach leaves

Gremolata (leftover from Tuesday's dinner)

1. Combine the lentils, tomatoes and spinach leaves in a serving bowl and drizzle with the gremolata to serve.

DINNER

Spaghetti with a creamy artichoke sauce

Under 700 calories

People who are new to veganism can find they miss creamy sauces, but you'll find this a great alternative. You won't use all the sauce (made from the soft cheese and artichokes) tonight, so save the rest in the fridge for lunch later in the week.

150g linguine

1 x 255g tub 'Free From' soft
   cheese

1 x 280g jar of artichoke hearts,
   drained and thinly sliced

Pepper, to taste

Zest of 1 lemon

TO SERVE

Small bunch of parsley,
   chopped

80g pine nuts

1. Cook the pasta according to the packet instructions.

2. Meanwhile, make the sauce. Mash the 'Free From' cheese, artichoke hearts, a lot of cracked black pepper and the lemon zest together. The 'sauce' will be quite thick at this stage. Set half aside in a covered bowl in the fridge for lunch tomorrow.

3. Toast the pine nuts in a dry pan for a few minutes, until fragrant, shaking the pan every now and then to stop them burning.

4. When the pasta is cooked through, drain, then return to the pan. Add half of the sauce and heat through until the cream cheese becomes slightly runnier. Save the other half for lunch later in the week. Serve the pasta scattered with the parsley and pine nuts.

The chia seeds for breakfast tomorrow need to be prepared tonight, and the strawberries need to be taken out of the freezer so they are defrosted by morning – see steps 1 and 2 on page 192.

BREAKFAST

Berry and vanilla chia pudding with a crunchy granola topping

Under 600 calories

The sweetness of the berries and vanilla, the creaminess of the chia pudding and the crunchiness of the topping go perfectly together. This breakfast is also very quick to make, as the majority of it will be made the night before. Chia puddings can also be made in Tupperware boxes and taken to work as an 'on the go' breakfast.

500ml hazelnut milk

60g chia seeds

2 tbsp agave nectar

1 tsp vanilla extract

110g frozen strawberries

Juice from ½ lime

60g homemade raspberry and cacao granola (see page 82)

---

1. Combine the hazelnut milk, chia seeds, agave and vanilla extract in a jar or bowl and set in the fridge for 15 minutes, then remove and mix again. Cover the bowl or jar with a lid or cling film and return to the fridge overnight.

2. Take the strawberries out of the freezer, squeeze over the lime juice and leave to defrost overnight.

3. In the morning, remove the chia pudding from the fridge, divide among two bowls, top with the strawberries and granola to serve.

LUNCH

Tartine with artichoke paté and pan-fried vegetables

Under 400 calories

The flavour of the artichokes in this tartine really comes through and complements the pan-fried vegetables well. Ideally, you need to cook the courgettes at the time so they are warm and crispy, but if you don't have cooking facilities during the day (e.g. because you're at work) then you can cook these in advance.

1 tsp olive oil	Artichoke sauce (leftover from
1 garlic clove, minced	Wednesday's dinner)
1 courgette, thinly sliced	
2 slices of sourdough bread, toasted	

1. In a shallow frying pan, heat the olive oil and add the garlic and courgette. Fry for about 7 minutes, until the courgette is soft and cooked through.

2. Spread the sourdough toast with the artichoke paté and pile with the courgette slices.

DINNER

Coconut and tomato daal with a zesty mango salad

Under 700 calories; under 1,000 including naan

The creamy daal in this dish is perfectly offset by the zesty mango. Daal is a great vegan main dish, as the lentils give you a good source of protein.

FOR THE SALAD
1 small mango, cut into small
   chunks
1 x 198g tin sweetcorn, drained
   and rinsed
2 tomatoes, cut into small
   chunks
1 bunch of coriander, chopped
Juice of 1 lime

FOR THE DAAL
½ tsp olive oil
1 white onion, diced
2 garlic cloves, diced
1 carrot, diced
1 tsp mustard seeds

1 tsp turmeric
1 tsp cumin seeds
Large knob of root ginger,
   finely grated
1 x 400g tin chopped tomatoes
80g dried black lentils, rinsed
100ml coconut cream (if you
   have more in the tin then
   freeze in a sealable bag or
   container for another meal)

TO SERVE (OPTIONAL)
Vegan naan breads (tortillas are
   OK if you are unable to find
   naans)

---

1. To make the salad, mix all the ingredients together. Set half the salad aside for lunch tomorrow.

2. Next, make the daal. Heat the olive oil in a saucepan and add the onion, garlic and carrot. Cover the pan and sweat the vegetables over a medium heat until soft, about 5 minutes.

3. Add the mustard, turmeric, cumin and ginger and stir well until the vegetable mixture is well coated with the spices.

4. Add the chopped tomatoes and black lentils. Using the tomato tin, fill it with water and add this to the saucepan, too.

5. Simmer for about 30 minutes, with the lid on, until the lentils have swollen and taken on much of the water and are cooked through. If the daal starts to dry out, add more water.

6. When the sauce is looking quite thick, add the coconut cream and mix thoroughly to combine.

7. Warm the naan in the oven according to the packet instructions, if using.

8. Serve the daal with the salad and warm naan.

BREAKFAST

Peanut butter and frozen banana smoothie

Under 300 calories

Using frozen bananas for this recipe makes the smoothie really cold and refreshing. The addition of dates and peanut butter makes it deliciously sweet too. This recipe is quite thick, so you may want to add some extra water or hazelnut milk if you prefer a thinner smoothie.

500ml hazelnut milk	4 tsp peanut butter
2 frozen bananas (from the freezer)	2 medjool dates

1. Put all the ingredients in a blender and blitz together for a few minutes until the smoothie becomes quite frothy.

2. If it is too thick, add extra water.

3. Pour into two glasses to serve.

LUNCH

Quinoa mango salad

Under 300 calories

Using leftovers from dinner yesterday means this recipe is incredibly quick to throw together. It is so colourful and pretty, and with the quinoa filling it is a good source of protein and slow-release carbohydrate.

120g quinoa
Mango salad (leftover from
   Thursday's dinner)

---

1. Cook the quinoa according to the packet instructions. Drain, then transfer to a large bowl and leave to cool. Stir the mango salad through the quinoa and serve.

DINNER

'Beany' chow

Under 800 calories

This recipe is a twist on a traditional South African dish called 'Bunny chow', consisting of a hollowed-out crusty loaf of bread filled with lamb or chicken curry – not rabbit as the name suggests. This makes the roll deliciously soft as it soaks up all the juices. In this version, the meat is replaced with beans for a vegan protein alternative.

1 tbsp olive oil

2 garlic cloves, minced

2 spring onions, thinly sliced

1 tbsp tomato purée

2 tsp chilli flakes (or more if you like it spicy!)

1 x 400g tin butter beans (keep the juices)

1 tsp salt

12 cherry tomatoes

1 tsp white wine vinegar

225g sundried tomatoes

TO SERVE

2 crusty wholemeal bread rolls

A handful of flat-leaf parsley, finely chopped

Tomato hummus, leftover from Sunday's dinner

Pepper, to taste

1. Preheat the oven to 150°C/130°C fan/300°F/gas mark 2.

2. In a pan over a medium heat, add the olive oil, garlic and spring onions and cook for a few minutes until soft.

3. Stir in the tomato purée, and chilli flakes.

4. Tip the beans with their juices and the salt into the pan over a medium heat and bring to the boil. Simmer for 5 minutes.

5. Add the tomatoes, white wine vinegar and sundried tomatoes and simmer for 10 minutes, until the sauce is really nice and thick.

6. For the last 5 minutes of the sauce thickening, heat the bread rolls in the oven.

7. When you remove the bread rolls from the oven, use a knife to cut around the top and remove the insides. Pile the stew into the middle of the bread rolls, and serve the removed bread on the side to 'mop up' any stew that may spill out.

8. Serve the bread rolls topped with parsley, hummus and pepper.

Recipes: Week 5

N.B. Each meal serves two people
unless otherwise stated.

SHOPPING LIST

Dairy alternatives

☐ 1 x 250g pot of coconut yoghurt

☐ 1 litre soya milk

Fruit and vegetables

☐ 1 white onion

☐ 1 red onion

☐ 75g new potatoes

☐ 1 sweet potato

☐ 2 red peppers

☐ 2 tomatoes

☐ 8 plum tomatoes

☐ 1 aubergine

☐ 2 courgettes

☐ 4 portobello mushrooms

☐ 100g green beans

☐ 200g blueberries

☐ 2 bananas

☐ 4 apricots

Dried store foods

☐ 2 x 400ml tins coconut milk

☐ 1 x 198g tin sweetcorn

Other

☐ 40g massaman curry paste

☐ 200g extra-firm tofu

☐ 10g dried crushed lavender

Fresh herbs

☐ Coriander*

☐ Basil*

*You may not need to buy these if you have leftovers from previous weeks.

MENU

	Breakfast	Lunch	Dinner
Saturday	Vegan French toast 'pockets' with blueberries and cinnamon	Sweet potato, corn and coconut soup	Ratatouille-stuffed mushrooms with a pearl barley salad
Sunday	Pancakes with apricots, lavender, coconut yoghurt and agave	Sourdough bruschetta	Tofu massaman curry

BREAKFAST

Vegan French toast 'pockets' with blueberries and cinnamon

Under 450 calories

These French toasts have the fruit stuffed inside them, so the whole toast is bursting with flavour when you cut into them. You can always mix up the fruit for variety – raspberries or strawberries are delicious, too!

FOR THE FRENCH TOAST 'POCKETS'
2 slices of wholemeal bread, cut 3cm thick
150g blueberries, plus 50g extra to serve
240ml soya milk
2 tbsp plain flour
1 tsp maple syrup, plus extra to serve
1 tsp vanilla extract
½ tsp salt
Pinch of grated nutmeg
1 banana
125g coconut yoghurt, to serve

1. Cut a slit into the longest side of each piece of bread to make a pocket.

2. Use your finger to stuff the blueberries inside, dividing them equally between the slices. Be careful – you don't want to tear the bread.

3. Add the soya milk, flour, maple syrup, vanilla extract, salt, nutmeg and banana to a blender and blitz together until completely smooth, then pour the mixture into a shallow bowl.

4. Heat a non-stick griddle or frying pan over a medium heat. Dip the bread slices into the soya milk mixture and transfer to the hot pan, then cook for about 5 minutes on each side until browned all over. Serve piled high with a dollop of coconut yoghurt, the extra blueberries and a drizzle of maple syrup.

LUNCH

Sweet potato, corn and coconut soup

Under 750 calories

This soup is very quick to make, as everything goes straight into one pot. I like it smooth, but you can leave it chunky if you prefer. The coriander on the top gives a lovely bit of colour contrast with the orange of the soup.

FOR THE SOUP
1 tbsp olive oil
1 white onion, diced
1 sweet potato, peeled and cut
   into small chunks
400ml vegetable stock, made
   from 1 stock cube

1 x 400ml tin coconut milk
1 x 198g tin sweetcorn

TO SERVE
Chopped coriander
Salt and pepper, to taste

1. Heat the olive oil in a pan over a low heat.

2. Add the onion and sweet potato and cook for about 5 minutes, until soft and slightly browned.

3. Add the stock, coconut milk and sweetcorn and simmer for 30 minutes, with the lid on, stirring occasionally to make sure nothing catches on the bottom.

4. Blend using a hand-held blender in the pan or transfer to a blender and blitz until smooth. Return to a clean pan to heat through, if needed, and serve hot with the chopped coriander on top and salt and pepper to taste.

DINNER

Ratatouille-stuffed mushrooms with a pearl barley salad

Under 700 calories

Ratatouille is a dish that originated in Nice, in the south of France. It is made with stewed vegetables, which make a perfect stuffing for mushrooms. Here you use portobello mushrooms, as they are large and flat, so are able to hold lots of the filling. The breadcrumbs give a lovely crunch; if you want to make you own you can follow the recipe on page 160.

FOR THE RATATOUILLE-
STUFFED MUSHROOMS
2 plum tomatoes
3 tbsp olive oil
1 red onion, diced
1 garlic clove, minced
1 aubergine, cut into small
   pieces
2 courgettes, 1 cut into small
   pieces, plus 1 sliced

1 red pepper, deseeded and
   diced
¼ tsp dark muscovado sugar
4 portobello mushrooms (2 per
   person)
50g breadcrumbs (see page
   160 to make your own)

TO SERVE
100g barley

Get ahead

If you like, you can soak the chia seeds for tomorrow's breakfast and leave them overnight in the fridge (see step 2 on page 211).

1. Preheat the oven to 180°C/160°C fan/350°F/gas mark 4.

2. Score a cross in the base of the tomatoes and place them in a heatproof bowl. Cover them with boiling water and set aside for 1 minute. Drain the water and set the tomatoes aside until cool enough to handle, then peel away the skins. Cut the tomatoes in half, scoop out the seeds and discard. Roughly chop the flesh.

3. In a pan over a low heat, heat 1 tablespoon of the olive oil then add the onion and garlic and cook over a gentle heat for 8 minutes, stirring occasionally, until golden-brown and very tender. Add the aubergine and courgette pieces for another 3 minutes.

4. Stir in the pepper, tomatoes and sugar, turn down the heat to very low, then cover and cook for 20 minutes until very soft.

5. Fill each mushroom with the ratatouille, top with the breadcrumbs and remaining olive oil and bake for 15–20 minutes, until the mushrooms are cooked through and soft and the breadcrumbs are crispy.

6. Cook the barley according to the packet instructions.

7. Heat the olive oil in a shallow frying pan and fry the courgette slices and the garlic, cooking the courgette on both sides for about 5 minutes on each side, until soft and browned.

8. Serve the barley with courgette and mushrooms on top.

BREAKFAST

Pancakes with apricots, lavender, coconut yoghurt and agave

Under 750 calories

Apricots and lavender give an amazing flavour combination which makes you feel like you are in the south of France. If you are struggling to buy lavender, the apricots will still be delicious if you leave it out.

FOR THE PANCAKES
30g chia seeds
4 tbsp water
1 banana
100g plain flour
150ml soya milk
1 tsp vegan butter

FOR THE STEWED FRUIT
4 apricots, halved and stoned
Agave nectar, for drizzling
10g dried crushed lavender
   (optional)

TO SERVE
125g coconut yoghurt

1. Preheat the oven to 180°C/160°C fan/350°F/gas mark 4.

2. Combine the chia seeds and water, and leave to sit in the fridge for at least 30 minutes to form a 'jelly'.

3. Start making the stewed fruit. Lay the apricots on a baking tray lined with baking parchment.

4. Fill the well of each half left by the stone with agave nectar and crushed lavender, if using, and bake for 10–15 minutes, until the fruit is caramelised.

5. While the fruit is cooking, make the pancake batter. Mash the banana in a bowl and put it into the blender, then add all the remaining pancake ingredients except the vegan butter and including the chia seed jelly. Blitz thoroughly until everything is combined. The batter should be nice and thick.

6. In a non-stick saucepan, heat the vegan butter over a medium heat. When hot and bubbling, scoop about ½ a cup of the batter (ideally using a small ladle if you have one) into the pan. Cook each pancake for about 2 minutes on each side; the outside should be darker in colour and bubbles will start to form in the mixture and it will hold your shape – this is how you know when they are ready to flip!

7. Repeat until you've used all the mixture; the recipe should make 6 small pancakes (3 each!). If at any time during the cooking you find the batter starts sticking, add more vegan butter.

8. Serve the pancakes stacked with the caramelised apricots and coconut yoghurt.

LUNCH

Sourdough bruschetta

Under 500 calories

Bruschetta is a classic Italian antipasto; it is traditional to rub the bread with a cut raw garlic clove to really bring out the flavour. This would also make a great snack or canapé for a dinner party.

6 plum tomatoes, finely chopped	(2 per person)
1 tbsp olive oil	1 garlic clove, cut in half
1 tsp white wine vinegar	Handful of basil leaves
4 slices of sourdough bread	Salt and pepper, to taste

1. Toss the tomatoes in a bowl with the oil, vinegar, salt and pepper.

2. Toast the sourdough and rub each slice with the cut sides of the raw garlic, so the garlicky flavour transfers well onto the toast.

3. Top the toast with the tomato mix and the basil leaves.

DINNER

Tofu massaman curry

Under 700 calories

This rich and mild Thai curry is an interpretation of a Persian dish. The massaman curry paste contains tamarind, which gives it a very particular, tangy taste. As this recipe contains potatoes, vegetables and protein, you don't need to serve it with any sides.

200g extra-firm tofu
40g massaman curry paste
1 x 400g tin coconut milk
75g new potatoes, chopped into bite-sized chunks
100g green beans, cut into thirds

1 red pepper, deseeded and diced
1 tbsp olive oil
50g raw peanuts, chopped
Coriander, chopped

1. Cut the tofu into small pieces, then wrap in a clean tea towel and press down gently to remove excess moisture.

2. Put the curry paste into a large saucepan and add the coconut milk, a small amount at a time (to stop it going lumpy), until all the coconut milk has been added.

3. Add the potatoes, then leave to simmer, about 10 minutes.

4. Add the green beans and pepper, and simmer for another 5 minutes until the veggies are tender and the curry sauce is starting to thicken.

5. Heat the oil in a frying pan and fry the tofu pieces on each side until slightly browned. Add the tofu to the curry mixture.

6. Toast the peanuts in a shallow frying pan over a low heat for about 5 minutes until aromatic, shaking the pan occasionally to make sure they don't burn. Make sure you watch the nuts closely.

7. Serve the curry, scattered with the peanuts and coriander.

Snacks

Apricot, almond and cashew balls

Makes 15
Calories per ball: Under 150

These energy balls have healthy fats from the nuts and a cheeky after-kick from the ginger.

300g cashew nuts
400g apricots, dried
Thumb-sized piece of fresh
   root ginger, grated
2 tbsp cashew butter (you can make your own, but I normally buy it. You can find it with peanut butter in most major supermarkets)
1½ tbsp coconut oil

1. Pulse the cashew nuts in a blender until they resemble a fine powder, then remove 100g of the powdered nuts and place them in a shallow bowl.

2. Add all of the remaining ingredients to the 200g of cashews in the blender bowl and blitz until smooth. If the mixture seems too thick, add some water, a tablespoon at a time.

3. Take a tablespoon of the mixture at a time and shape it into a ball, then roll each in the cashew nut powder until coated.

4. Store the balls in an airtight container in the fridge and eat within a few days (but mine never last that long!).

Date, cacao and coconut energy balls

Makes 15 balls
Calories per ball: Under 150

These indulgent snacks are delicious; the dates make them sticky while the raw cacao makes them feel like a real treat. They are so pretty too.

200g ground almonds	2½ tbsp almond butter
400g medjool dates	2 tbsp coconut oil
4 tbsp raw cacao powder	80g desiccated coconut

1. Blend all the ingredients together in a food processor, except the desiccated coconut, until smooth. If the mixture seems too thick, add some water, a tablespoon at a time.

2. Place the desiccated coconut in a shallow bowl.

3. Take a tablespoon of the mixture at a time and shape into a ball, then roll each in the coconut to coat.

4. Store in an airtight container in the fridge and eat within a few days.

No 'cook'ies

Makes 25
Calories per 'cook'ie: Under 100

These have slow-release energy from the oats, healthy fats from the seeds and natural sweetness from the dried fruit, so they make a great snack if you're peckish. N.B. for step 2, you will need a strong blender.

50g prunes	50g whole almonds
50g dates, stoned	150g chunky oats
1 banana	50g sunflower seeds
1 tbsp coconut oil	50g flame raisins (these are
1 tsp ground cinnamon	the nice big juicy ones!)
2 tbsp maple syrup	50g sesame seeds

1. Blitz the prunes, dates, banana, coconut oil, cinnamon and maple syrup together in a blender. Transfer the mixture from the blender to a large mixing bowl.

2. Blitz the almonds in the blender until they are roughly chopped (you don't need to clean the blender first). Beware: this makes a horrible noise! Tip them into the mixing bowl with the pruney paste.

3. Add the oats, sunflower seeds and raisins to the mixing bowl and stir all the ingredients together.

4. In the palm of your hand, take some mixture and shape into golf-ball-sized pieces. At this stage, they might be quite tricky to bind together.

5. Tip the sesame seeds in a shallow bowl. Roll each ball in the sesame seeds then roll again in the palms of your hands. With the sesame seed 'coating', the cookie will start to bind together.

6. After you have finished all the cookies, pop them in the fridge to set. Store in an airtight container in the fridge and eat within a few days.

Sweet sesame roasted nuts

Makes 6 servings
Calories per serving: under 250

This snack is so easy to make and will really impress anyone who tries it. The perfect snack to put into a little Tupperware box in your bag for a pick-me-up on the go.

280g whole almonds	Scant ½ tsp cayenne pepper
2 tbsp agave syrup	35g sesame seeds
¼ tsp salt	

1. Preheat the oven to 170°C/150°C fan/325°F/gas mark 3. Line a baking tray with baking parchment.

2. Mix all the ingredients together in a bowl so that the nuts are well coated.

3. Tip out the nuts onto the baking tray and roast in the oven for 10 minutes.

4. Once toasted, remove from the oven and leave to cool fully, then gently break up the almonds. Store in an airtight container for up to a week.

Tortilla chips with a cashew and roasted pepper dip

Serves 8
Calories: Under 300

I love this recipe – the combination of the crispy tortilla chips and the creamy cashew dip is heaven. You get healthy fats and protein from the nuts and carbohydrate from the tortillas, balancing the snack.

1 red pepper, halved and de-seeded	1 teaspoon salt to taste
2 tsp olive oil	4 flour tortillas (alternatively, you can buy plain corn tortilla chips instead of making your own)
1 clove of garlic, minced	
200g cashews	
½ lemon, juiced	
175ml water	Salt and pepper to taste

1. Preheat the oven to 180°C/160°C fan/350°F/gas mark 4.

2. Drizzle the halved red pepper with olive oil and top evenly with the crushed garlic, then roast for 20 minutes until soft.

3. Meanwhile, soak the cashews in water for 30 minutes, then drain and place in a blender.

4. When you remove the red pepper from the oven, put into a sandwich bag while hot. This will loosen the skin. Peel the skin away and discard, so you are left with the flesh only.

5. Put the red pepper flesh into the blender with the nuts, lemon juice, 175ml water, the salt to taste, and blend until smooth. Spoon into a bowl.

6. Cut the tortillas into eight wedges each, then spread them out on a baking sheet in a single layer.

7. Bake the tortilla chips for 6 minutes, then remove from the oven, turn them over and cook on the other side for another 6 minutes – they should be crispy and just beginning to colour.

8. Serve with the red pepper dip and enjoy!

Sourdough fingers with a hot artichoke dip

Serves 4

Calories per serving: Under 400

This dip is incredibly simple to make and really delicious. The artichoke gives it an unusual flavour and the tofu gives you a good hit of protein.

150g raw cashews (soaked in water 4–8 hours), drained and rinsed	60ml nut milk of choice
	1 handful of spinach
	150g artichoke hearts
150g silken tofu	1 bunch of chives
3 garlic cloves	Salt and pepper, to taste
Juice of 1 lemon	4 slices sourdough toast

1. Put the cashews, tofu, garlic, lemon juice, salt and pepper into a food processor and blitz to a paste.

2. With the food processor running, drizzle in the milk, using just enough to get the mixture to a creamy consistency, with a thickness like that of yoghurt.

3. Add the remaining ingredients and pulse until they are chopped and well mixed into the rest of the ingredients, but not smooth.

4. Transfer the dip into a saucepan and place over a medium heat, stirring constantly until warmed through. If it seems too thick for you, add a small amount of milk to prevent the dip drying out.

5. Serve with toasted sourdough fingers.

Kale crisps

Serves 4
Calories: under 100 per serving

These couldn't be easier to make and always really impress a crowd – they are a great healthy alternative to crisps before a meal with friends, but they are also a nice accompaniment to a meal.

4 large handfuls of kale, tough stalks removed
1 tsp chilli flakes (I buy these in bags and keep them in the freezer – very handy!)
OR nutritional yeast (to give them a 'cheesy' flavour)
1 tsp olive oil
A very generous amount of cracked black pepper

1. Preheat the oven to 180°C/160°C fan/350°F/gas mark 4.

2. Wash and dry the kale very thoroughly – it is important that there is not too much moisture on the kale or it will not get crispy. Tip the leaves into a clean tea towel and pat dry.

3. Spread the kale evenly on a baking tray.

4. Sprinkle with the chilli flakes or nutritional yeast, olive oil and pepper.

5. Bake in the oven for 10 minutes until crispy.

Garlic and herb celeriac wedges

Serves 8
Calories per serving: under 100

Celeriac is an unusual flavour, and many people don't eat it because they don't know how to. And you don't need to limit to using it in meals — it works well as a snack also.

---

1 celeriac, peeled and cut into
  wedges
2 tbsp dried oregano
2 garlic cloves, crushed

Salt and pepper, to taste
2 tbsp olive oil
5 sprigs of rosemary

---

1. Preheat the oven to 200°C/180°C fan/400°F/gas mark 6.

2. Fill a pan with cold water and add the celeriac. Bring to the boil and allow to bubble away for 5 minutes.

3. Once cooked, drain the celeriac wedges and wait for a few minutes for the steam to evaporate so that they are really dry before adding the oregano, garlic, salt and pepper and mix well.

4. Meanwhile, heat the oil in a baking tray in the oven for a few minutes. When the oil is hot, remove the tray from the oven and add the coated wedges to the tray. Toss well to ensure they are well coated in the hot oil.

5. Top with the rosemary sprigs and return the tray to the oven to cook for 35–40 minutes.

Popcorn with chilli flakes and nutritional yeast

Serves 2
Calories per serving: 250

Popcorn is a brilliant snack – a really nice way to kick back in the evening with a film. Adding nutritional yeast and chilli gives it a little 'kick' and makes it taste quite 'cheesy.'

2 tbsp olive oil	1 tsp chilli flakes
50g corn kernels	Salt and pepper, to taste
2 tbsp nutritional yeast	

1. Heat the oil in a saucepan on a medium-high heat.

2. Put the corn kernels into the oil and cover the pan, leaving the lid slightly ajar.

3. The corn should begin popping soon. While popping, gently shake the pan by moving it back and forth over the burner.

4. When the popping slows to a few seconds between each pop, remove from the heat. To serve, sprinkle over the nutritional yeast, chilli flakes, salt and pepper, then toss to combine.

Trail Mix

Makes 8 servings
Calories per serving: under 300

You can really throw together any combination of nuts and dried fruit for a trail mix, but this is my favourite.

100g cashews	100g vegan chocolate chips
100g salted almonds	(or vegan chocolate, cut into
100g dried cranberries	small chunks)

1. Mix all the ingredients together in a small bowl to combine, then store in an airtight container for up to one week.

Extra Information

FAQs about healthy eating

IS SUGAR ADDICTIVE?

There are many claims that sugar, like alcohol and drugs, is addictive; this is a theory called 'the sugar addiction hypothesis'. Like some drugs, sugar is rapidly absorbed into the body and stimulates the pleasure centres in the brain (through neurotransmitters, dopamine and opioids) and so we can crave more. However, there is not yet evidence that sugar causes withdrawal in the same way that other addictive substances can. Furthermore, many things light up pleasure centres in the brain, such as photos of your family or friends, and this doesn't necessarily make those things addictive. Many of the studies investigating this hypothesis are being conducted using animals, not humans, so we cannot draw direct comparisons between the two. The jury is very much still out!

SHOULD I GO ON A 'DETOX' DIET?

Detox diets and products claim to help rid your body of unwanted substances called toxins. Detox diets tend to be highly restrictive, and detox products are often very expensive. Sometimes people feel better after doing a detox, but this is usually because you are restricting calories (which can make you feel good in the short term), drinking lots of water and not smoking or drinking alcohol.

If your liver and kidneys are working well, your body is capable of doing all the detoxing that it needs. In fact, every time you go to the loo you are detoxing, as you are getting rid of waste from the body! If you feel run down, make sure you get a good night's sleep, drink lots of water, reduce your consumption of processed (fast) food, eat lots of vegetables and cut down on smoking and drinking alcohol. That's all the detoxing your body needs.

IS BUYING ORGANIC BETTER FOR MY HEALTH?

Ingredients are termed organic when the food has been produced without the use of artificial chemicals, such as pesticides or fertilisers. Many people choose organic food for its perceived nutritional or environmental benefits. Whether or not organic food is better for health has been a booming area of research, as some studies have looked at the nutritional composition of both organically and conventionally produced crops and found very few differences! Some people choose to buy organic food because they believe it is safer and more nutritious than food produced by modern farming methods, but at present the scientific evidence does not support this. It is, of course, your choice, but because organic food is more expensive, if you choose to shop this way and find that the cost reduces your intake of fruits and vegetables, you may in fact be making your diet less healthy!

WHAT ARE SUPERFOODS AND SHOULD I EAT THEM?

Superfoods are foods that are high in some nutrients and are hailed as the magic cure, giving you more energy and/or preventing or curing disease. However, a superfood is just a marketing term – there is nothing scientific or evidence-based behind this claim. The really unusual ingredients are often very expensive, and to get the required nutrients from them, you need a lot of them. For example, pink Himalayan sea salt is often called a 'superfood' for its high magnesium content, but to reach your daily requirement of magnesium you would need to eat 2kg per day of the stuff – and that much salt would be detrimental to your body. If you can afford superfoods and you want to include them in your diet, go ahead and do so in moderation, but you don't need expensive, trendy foods in your diet to be healthy.

IS COCONUT OIL GOOD FOR ME?

Coconut oil has had a lot of good press lately for its perceived health benefits. We are in such a craze about this ingredient that, according to the UN's Food and Agriculture Organization (FAO), global demand is growing at 10 per cent per year and the global market for coconut water hit $2.26 billion in 2016. It seems our appetite for coconuts is insatiable. But why?

Coconut is a plant fat, so many assumed it was good for us. However, coconut oil is about 86 per cent saturated (bad) fat, which is even higher than butter! For a while, some people thought that the fat in coconut oil was better for us than other saturated fats, but so far we don't have a good, science-based answer for that. But we do know that replacing saturated fats with unsaturated (good) fats is an effective way to reduce bad cholesterol levels and lowers the risk of heart disease and strokes. So, for now, if you like a little bit of coconut oil, use it sparingly as you would have used butter. Opt instead for nuts, seeds, nut butters and other vegetable oils to provide you with the fat you need in your diet.

Where can I go for more information?

The Vegan Society

Website: www.vegansociety.com
How it can help you: The Vegan Society has lots of advice and support for people wanting to step out into a vegan lifestyle, such as hints and tips for food shopping and regular blog articles about vegan restaurants, cafes and new foods.

People for the Ethical Treatment of Animals (PETA)

Website: www.peta.org.uk
How it can help you: PETA is a charity that has been instrumental in setting up 'Veganuary', and therefore is very supportive of trying 30 days of vegan living. It has lots of information about ethical companies, recipes and even an online shop. You can even order a 'vegan starter kit'.

British Dietetic Association

Website: www.bda.uk.com
How it can help you: This is the trade union for dietitians in the UK. It contains evidence-based dietary information which you can trust, all written by registered dietitians. You can download fact sheets on veganism and many different vitamins and minerals, including those mentioned earlier in this book, such as iron and iodine.

Freelance Dietitians

Website: http://freelancedietitians.org
How it can help you: This website provides contact details for freelance dietitians around the United Kingdom. Dietitians are the only profession that is tightly regulated by an ethical code to provide you with safe, effective and evidence-based information. If you want tailored nutrition advice, this would be a great place to start.

Association for Nutrition (AfN)

Website: www.associationfornutrition.org
How it can help you: AfN is a registered charity that holds the UK Voluntary Register of Nutritionists (UKVRN), accrediting nutritionists with a certain academic qualification either at undergraduate or postgraduate level. It aims to protect and benefit the public by defining and advancing standards of evidence-based practice across the field of nutrition and at all levels within the workforce.

If you want to see a nutritionist, the AfN register will provide you with the resources to access qualified professionals.

London Vegan Meetup

Website: www.meetup.com/londonvegan
How it can help you: London Vegan Meetup holds regular events for like-minded people to get together to enjoy vegan food. You don't have to be a vegan to go to their events, but you will only be eating vegan food at them! If you don't live in London, look on the Meetup website to see if you can find similar groups to join.

References

Craig, W.J. (2009), 'Health effects of vegan diets', *American Society for Nutrition*: 89 (5).

Davey, G.K., Spencer, E.A., Appleby P.N., Allen, N.E., Knox, K.H. and Key, T.J. (2002), 'EPIC–Oxford: lifestyle characteristics and nutrient intakes in a cohort of 33 883 meat-eaters and 31 546 non meat-eaters in the UK', *Public Health Nutrition*: 6 (3).

Fuhrman, J and Ferreri, D.M. (2010), 'Fueling the Vegetarian (Vegan) Athlete', *Current Sports, Medicine Reports:* 9 (4).

Jenkins, D.J.A., Kendall, C.W.C., Marchie, A., Jenkins, A.L., Augustin, L.S.A., Ludwig, D.S., Barnard, N.D. and Anderson J.W. (2003), 'Type 2 diabetes and the vegetarian diet', *American Journal of Clinical Nutrition*; 8 (3).

Krajčovičová-Kudláčková M.A, Bučková K.B., Klimeš I.B.,Šeboková E.B. (2003), 'Iodine Deficiency in Vegetarians and Vegans', *Annals of Nutrition and Metabolism*; 47.

McDougall, J., Bruce, B., Spiller, G., Westerdahl, J. McDougall, M. (2002), 'Effects of a Very Low-Fat, Vegan Diet in Subjects with Rheumatoid Arthritis', *The Journal of Alternative and Complementary Medicine*: 8 (1).

Messier, S.P., Loeser, R.F., Miller, G.D. Morgan, T.M, Rejeski, W.J., Sevick, M.A., Ettinger, W.H. Pahor, M. and Williamson, J.D. (2004), 'Exercise and dietary weight loss in overweight and obese older adults with knee osteoarthritis: the Arthritis, Diet, and Activity Promotion Trial', *Arthritis & Rheumatology*: 50 (5).

Sharma, R., Biedenharn, K.R., Fedor, J.M. and Agarwal, A. (2013), 'Lifestyle factors and reproductive health: taking control of your fertility', *Reproductive Biology and Endocrinology*. Available from: https://rbej.biomedcentral.com/articles/10.1186/ 1477-7827-11-66 (Accessed on: 12 September 2017).

Williams, C., (2002). 'Nutritional quality of organic food: shades of grey or shades of green?', *Proceedings of the Nutrition Society*: 61.

General Index

A
antioxidants 9, 16
arthritis 16

B
blood pressure 9
BMI (Body Mass Index) 9
bone health 12, 22

C
calcium 12, 20, 22-3
calories 3, 12-13, 20
cancers 3, 10-11
carbohydrates 4, 12, 13, 14, 15, 16, 18
cardiovascular disease 3, 9
cholesterol 9, 21
coconut oil 231

D
dairy foods 2, 7, 12, 13, 19, 22, 24, 26
    alternatives 3, 13, 17
detox diet 229-30
diabetes 3, 11

F
fats 13, 20, 23, 231
    sources 20-1
fertility 16

fibre 3, 6, 9, 10, 16
    daily intake 18
fish 4, 19, 26
flavourings 4
FODMAPs 7, 14
fruit & veg 4, 7, 9, 10, 11, 14, 16, 17-18

H
health, and plant-based diet 3
heart attacks 9
heart health 9-10

I
IBS (Irritable Bowel Syndrome) 14-15
iodine 20, 25-6
iron deficiency 14

M
meat 2, 3, 4, 10, 11, 13, 14, 15, 19, 24, 25, 26
minerals 4, 13, 17, 24, 25

O
organic foods 230
osteoarthritis 16

P
processed foods 3, 6, 10, 11, 230
proteins 13, 19–20, 23

S
sugar, and addiction 229
superfoods 230–1

V
vegan diet
  and animal products 5, 7
  and children 7–8
  benefits the heart 9–10, 21
  dietary/health benefits 3, 6, 9–11,
    16, 21
  and eating out 5–6
  facts and myths re health 3,
    9–16

ingredients 10
mental health 15
and omnivores 9, 10
and other diets 7
practicalities of taking up 5–7
preparing meals 4–5
reasons for taking up 2–5
and weight loss 12–13
vegetables, *also see* fruit
  seasonal 4
vitamins 3, 4, 8, 10, 13, 14, 17, 20,
  24, 25

Recipe Index

A

A Lebanese feast: imam, hummus, flatbread and a nutty kale salad 86

Almond butter and fig porridge 188

Apple and ginger bircher muesli 150

Apricot, almond and cashew balls 216

Apricot, blueberry and hazelnut bircher muesli 118

Aromatic crispy tofu stir-fry 60

Artichoke and broad bean salad with a tahini dressing 98

Aubergine katsu curry 131

B

Banana, fig and pear muffins 168

Banana, maple syrup and pecan porridge 72

'Beany' chow 198

Beetroot sliders 116

Berry and vanilla chia pudding with a crunchy granola topping 192

Berry blast smoothie 102

Borscht 130

Broad bean, asparagus and mint tartine 84

Butternut squash bisque 42

C

Cacao, date and banana smoothie 146

Caponata-inspired spaghetti 94

Chia pudding with coconut, pomegranate and pistachios 96

Chilli non-carne with hummus and avocado 50

Coconut and tomato daal with a zesty mango salad 194

Crispy tofu, hummus and avocado pitta 64

Currant tea loaf with homemade jam 46

D

Date, cacao and coconut energy balls 217

F

Falafel wrap 69

Fennel and white bean soup 92

Fennel, white bean and courgetti salad with tahini dressing 114

G

Gado-gado with quinoa 151

Garlic and herb celeriac wedges 225

H

Hot aubergine pockets 136
Hummus and grilled courgette wrap
185

I

Indian-spiced tomato and white
bean salad 147

K

Kale crisps 224
Korean quinoa bowls 104

L

Layered summer fruit parfait with
coconut yoghurt and granola 140
Leftover beetroot sliders with
buckwheat tabbouleh 119
Lemon and pea risotto with roasted
asparagus spears 120
Lentil salad with gremolata 189
Linguine with a mushroom and
chestnut sauce 74

M

Mango and coconut chia pudding 68
Mango and coconut smoothie 53
Mango, tomato and basil salad 155
Mediterranean-inspired sandwiches
73
Mexican brunch bowl 40
Multi-grain porridge 106
Mushroom and rocket polenta tart
with gremolata 186

N

No 'cook'ies 218
Nutty quinoa salad with fresh veggies
and mustard vinaigrette 108

P

Pancakes with apricots, lavender,
coconut yoghurt and agave 210
Pancakes with stewed autumn fruits
and coconut yoghurt 90
Peanut butter and frozen banana
smoothie 196
Pear and date bircher muesli 184
Popcorn with chilli flakes and
nutritional yeast 226
Porridge with vanilla poached plums
158

Q

Quinoa bowl – baked asparagus,
cherry tomatoes, peppers with
hummus and balsamic glaze 70
Quinoa bowl – harissa-roasted
aubergine, garlic mushrooms,
spinach and hummus 148
Quinoa granola with dried
raspberries and cacao nibs 82
Quinoa mango salad 197
Quinoa-stuffed peppers with
Moroccan flavours 160

R

Rainbow wild rice salad with a tangy
dressing 103
Ratatouille-stuffed mushrooms with
a pearl barley salad 208
Raw carrot gazpacho 170

Raw date, pecan and walnut breakfast bars 128
Red Thai butter bean curry with wild rice 100
Roast vegetable and polenta tart with kale and walnut pesto 56
Roasted vegetable and pesto pasta salad 59
Rösti topped with rocket and mashed avo 134

S
Savoury oatmeal with sautéed mushrooms and thyme 44
'Shepherd-less' pie with sweet potato mash 110
Smashed avocado and spiced chickpeas on toast 112
Sourdough bruschetta 212
Sourdough fattoush with butter beans 141
Sourdough fingers with a hot artichoke dip 223
Sourdough toast with peanut butter and homemade chia jam 58
Spaghetti with a creamy artichoke sauce 190
Spiced carrot, date and lentil salad 49
Spicy sweetcorn fritters with avocado and coriander 174
Spinach crepes with a pepper filling 156
Strawberry and soya breakfast smoothie 180
Sweet potato and chickpea curry with a spiced tomato salad 143

Sweet potato, corn and coconut soup 206
Sweet potato falafel with jewelled couscous 66
Sweet potato 'Tex-Mex' salad 54
Sweet sesame roasted nuts 220
Sweetcorn and bean wrap 181

T
Tamarind and coconut curry with quinoa 182
Tartine with artichoke paté and pan-fried vegetables 193
Tempeh kebabs with a peanut dipping sauce 138
Toasted muesli with dried fruit and nuts 62
Toasted spiced chickpea salad 176
Tofu massaman curry 213
Tortilla chips with a cashew and roasted pepper dip 221
Trail mix 227
Tropical popical smoothie 154
Turkish tomato salad with coconut haydari 159

V
Vegan French toast 'pockets' with blueberries and cinnamon 204
Vegan pizza with roasted tomato hummus 178
Vegan quinoa sushi 152
Vegan sausages with truffle mash 172

Acknowledgements

I've met a lot of very knowledgeable people who have given me advice about nutrition and the vegan diet, during my studies to become a dietitian and since I qualified. I must give a special mention to everyone I met at King's College, University of London, without whom I would not know half of what I do now, and the brilliant NHS dietitians I have worked with since, who teach me more every day.

Secondly, to all those people who gave me the inspiration to write this book, particularly Alice and Rory, who were the first of my friends to try out 'going vegan'. To my patients, who inspired the FAQs section – every question you ask is important, and we can both learn from them.

Thirdly, to all the people who made this dream a reality. My friend and editor, Emily Barrett, for her patience, insight and amazing eye for detail. And: Katie Horrocks, for getting the book safely to print; Helen Ewing and Debbie Holmes for overseeing the shoot; Vincent Whiteman for taking the photos; Laurie Perry for preparing the food; and Rebecca Newport for the props – the photos are something to be proud of!

And finally, to you! If you have enjoyed the recipes, learned anything from the introduction or enjoyed flipping through the photographs, please get in touch. I'd love to hear all your stories.

About the author

Catherine Kidd is a cook, foodie and dietitian. She began cooking with her mother at home as soon as she was able to hold a wooden spoon, so becoming a dietitian after leaving school was an obvious next step, allowing her to combine her interest in health and wellbeing with food. She did her masters degree in nutrition, completing her dissertation examining the effects of a vegan diet on the heart, for which she received the Drummond Award from the British Nutrition Foundation for 'excellence in science communication'. *30 Days Vegan* is her first book. She works both privately and for the NHS as a dietitian.

To contact Catherine:

Facebook: Catherine Kidd Nutrition
Instagram: catherinekiddnutrition
Twitter: CatherineKiddRD
Website: www.catherinekiddnutrition.com

STORE CUPBOARD ESSENTIALS

Oils, vinegars and sauces

- [ ] Olive oil
- [ ] Coconut oil
- [ ] Soy sauce
- [ ] White wine vinegar
- [ ] Tomato ketchup
- [ ] Balsamic vinegar
- [ ] Rice vinegar
- [ ] Yellow miso paste
- [ ] Horseradish sauce
- [ ] Pomegranate molasses
- [ ] Truffle-infused olive oil (optional – but not as expensive as you would expect and you can buy it easily from most supermarkets)

Fruit and nuts

- [ ] Capers
- [ ] Dried apricots
- [ ] Medjool dates
- [ ] Sesame seeds
- [ ] Linseeds
- [ ] Chia seeds
- [ ] Pistachio nuts
- [ ] Walnuts
- [ ] Pecans
- [ ] Peanuts
- [ ] Hazelnuts
- [ ] Flaked almonds

Carbohydrate staples

- [ ] Plain flour
- [ ] Rolled oats
- [ ] Quinoa
- [ ] Couscous
- [ ] Barley
- [ ] Buckwheat
- [ ] Dried wholewheat linguine/ spaghetti
- [ ] Dried penne (or other short pasta)
- [ ] Polenta/cornmeal
- [ ] Rice of your choice
- [ ] Risotto rice
- [ ] Wild rice
- [ ] Dried rice noodles

Herbs, flavourings and spices

- [ ] Agave nectar
- [ ] Maple syrup
- [ ] Balsamic glaze
- [ ] Tahini
- [ ] Thai red curry paste (buy the best one you can find, as this will have a huge impact on the flavour of the dishes you use it in)
- [ ] Harissa paste
- [ ] Tabasco sauce
- [ ] Sriracha sauce
- [ ] Za'atar
- [ ] Cardamom pods
- [ ] Turmeric
- [ ] Mustard seeds
- [ ] Mixed spice
- [ ] Salt
- [ ] Pepper and black peppercorns
- [ ] Paprika
- [ ] Chilli flakes
- [ ] Cumin – ground
- [ ] Dried oregano
- [ ] Dried rosemary
- [ ] Dried bay leaves
- [ ] Cinnamon – ground and sticks
- [ ] Coriander – ground and seeds
- [ ] Ground allspice
- [ ] Cardamom pods
- [ ] Moroccan spice mix
- [ ] Tomato purée
- [ ] Nutmeg – whole
- [ ] Cacao powder
- [ ] Vanilla extract

Other

- [ ] Vegetable stock cubes
- [ ] Nutritional yeast flakes
- [ ] Peanut butter (if you can, buy a good brand without added sugar)
- [ ] Dark muscovado sugar
- [ ] Soya protein powder (or other vegan alternative, if preferred)
- [ ] Baking powder
- [ ] Bran flakes

- [ ] Dry sherry (optional)
- [ ] Vegan yeast extract, e.g. Marmite/Vegemite
- [ ] Strong English breakfast tea bags

For the freezer

- [ ] Sliced sourdough bread (or other bread if you prefer!)
- [ ] Wholemeal pitta breads
- [ ] Peas
- [ ] Broad beans
- [ ] Root ginger (buy fresh, chop into knobs and freeze)

For the fridge

- [ ] Olive oil spread/vegan butter (make sure you check the nutrition information, as many margarines contain buttermilk)

Other

- [ ] Tin foil
- [ ] Cling film
- [ ] Wooden skewers
- [ ] Tupperware boxes (if you want to take lunch to work)

SHOPPING LIST WEEK 1

Dairy alternatives

- [ ] 1 litre coconut milk
- [ ] 250g pot of coconut yoghurt
- [ ] 1 litre hazelnut milk
- [ ] 1 litre soya milk

Fruit and vegetables

- [ ] 3 white onions
- [ ] 4 red onions
- [ ] 6 sweet potatoes
- [ ] 550g cherry tomatoes
- [ ] 5 plum tomatoes
- [ ] 5 avocados
- [ ] 2 courgettes
- [ ] 1 pak choi*
- [ ] 100g tenderstem broccoli*
- [ ] 100g baby corn*
- [ ] 100g sugar snap peas*
- [ ] 3 red peppers
- [ ] 200g asparagus
- [ ] 120g bag of rocket
- [ ] 150g kale
- [ ] 1 celery head (keep 3 sticks for week 2)
- [ ] 1 butternut squash
- [ ] 1 leek
- [ ] 1 carrot
- [ ] 620g chestnut mushrooms
- [ ] small box pomegranate seeds
- [ ] 1 chilli pepper
- [ ] 4 small-medium bananas
- [ ] 500g bag of frozen mango chunks
- [ ] 500g blackberries (fresh or frozen)
- [ ] 200g fresh raspberries
- [ ] 3 limes
- [ ] 3 lemons

Carbohydrate staples

☐ 2 bread rolls

☐ 8 flour tortilla wraps
(freeze the 4 left over
separately, laid flat in large
sandwich bags)

Dried fruit, nuts and seeds

☐ 200g desiccated coconut

☐ 250g dried fruit and nut
mix **

☐ 350g dried mixed fruit

Other

☐ 1 x 435g tin refried beans

☐ 2 x 400g tins chickpeas

☐ 100g silken tofu

☐ 1 x 400g tin pinto beans

☐ 1 x 400g tin chopped
tomatoes

☐ 250g ready cooked puy
lentils

☐ 1 x 400g tin black beans

☐ 1 x 198g tin sweetcorn

☐ 500g firm tofu

☐ White wine of your choice
(at least 70ml)

Fresh herbs

☐ Coriander***

☐ Parsley***

☐ Mint***

☐ Thyme***

☐ Rosemary***

☐ Lemongrass stalk

*Often you can buy these
ingredients together in a stir-
fry pack, which is cheaper and
reduces waste

**If you want to make your
own fruit and nut mix, you
need to buy the following:

☐ 20g sesame seeds

☐ 50g sunflower seeds

☐ 20g linseeds

☐ 50g hazelnuts

☐ 50g dried sour cherries

☐ 20g chia seeds

☐ 40g sultanas

***I would suggest buying a
pot of these herbs rather than
a packet – they will keep for
longer and be cheaper in the
long run.

SHOPPING LIST WEEK 2

Dairy alternatives

- [ ] 250g pot coconut yoghurt (some to be used next week so keep in fridge!)
- [ ] 1 litre almond milk
- [ ] 1 litre hazelnut milk

Fruit and vegetables

- [ ] 3 white onions
- [ ] 6 red onions
- [ ] 1 sweet potato
- [ ] 6 spring onions
- [ ] 2 red peppers and 1 pepper of your choice
- [ ] 3 small pak choi (or 1-2 big ones!)
- [ ] 100g sugar snap peas
- [ ] 1 cauliflower
- [ ] 1 beetroot
- [ ] 3 medium avocados
- [ ] 2 bunches asparagus
- [ ] 4 tomatoes
- [ ] 100 cherry tomatoes
- [ ] 200g kale
- [ ] 3 celery sticks
- [ ] ½ cucumber
- [ ] 2 aubergines
- [ ] 2 large fennel bulbs
- [ ] 100g artichoke hearts (from the deli section)
- [ ] 200g wild mushrooms
- [ ] 80g pomegranate seeds (or leftover from week 1)
- [ ] 2 courgettes
- [ ] 1 broccoli head
- [ ] 1 x 198g tin pineapple chunks
- [ ] 2 limes
- [ ] 1 dessert apple
- [ ] 6 lemons
- [ ] 2 cooking apples
- [ ] 350g frozen mixed berries
- [ ] 4 small-medium bananas
- [ ] 4 dried apricots
- [ ] 30g blueberries

Carbohydrate staples

- [ ] 2 burger buns/ bread rolls
- [ ] 2 flatbreads
- [ ] 110g fresh breadcrumbs*

Dried store foods

- [ ] 1 x 400g tin coconut milk
- [ ] 2 x 400g tins butter beans
- [ ] 3 x 400g tins chickpeas
- [ ] 1 x 198g tin sweetcorn
- [ ] 1 x 400g tin chopped tomatoes
- [ ] 1 x 200g tin haricot beans
- [ ] 1 x 400g tin cannellini beans

Other

- [ ] 200g ready-cooked firm tofu
- [ ] 150g dried cranberries
- [ ] 250g pine nuts
- [ ] 150g sundried tomatoes
- [ ] 125g cacao nibs
- [ ] 30g freeze-dried raspberries (if you prefer, you can use other dried fruits)
- [ ] 50g dessicated coconut
- [ ] 2 lemongrass sticks

Fresh herbs

- [ ] Mint**
- [ ] Coriander**
- [ ] Chives
- [ ] Parsley**
- [ ] Dill

*Instead of buying breadcrumbs, you can make some (see page 160 for recipe)

**You may not need to buy these if you have leftovers from last week.

SHOPPING LIST WEEK 3

Dairy alternatives

- [ ] 1 litre hazelnut milk
- [ ] 1 litre almond milk

Fruit and vegetables

- [ ] 4 red onions
- [ ] 1 white onion
- [ ] 1 large potato
- [ ] 1 sweet potato
- [ ] 6 spring onions
- [ ] 600g cherry tomatoes
- [ ] 2 small cucumbers
- [ ] 4 avocados
- [ ] 300g spinach
- [ ] 3 red peppers
- [ ] 4 Romano peppers
- [ ] 1 little gem lettuce
- [ ] 125g bag of rocket
- [ ] 150g sundried tomatoes
- [ ] 150g artichoke hearts
- [ ] 3 aubergines
- [ ] 150g chestnut mushrooms
- [ ] 3 carrots
- [ ] 1 beetroot
- [ ] 1 courgette
- [ ] 100g green beans
- [ ] 4 plum tomatoes
- [ ] 1 very small red cabbage
- [ ] 4 limes
- [ ] 4 lemons
- [ ] 130g fresh pineapple chunks
- [ ] 6 plums
- [ ] 4 bananas
- [ ] 2 dessert apples
- [ ] 1 small mango
- [ ] 100g raspberries
- [ ] 100g strawberries

Dried store foods

- [ ] 2 x 400ml tins reduced-fat coconut milk
- [ ] 2 x 400g tins chickpeas
- [ ] 1 x 400g tin butter beans
- [ ] 1 x 227g tin chopped tomatoes

- ☐ 200g ready-to-eat quinoa lentil mix
- ☐ 110g preserved lemon

Other

- ☐ 400ml orange juice
- ☐ 3 sheets sushi nori
- ☐ Wasabi paste
- ☐ Pickled ginger
- ☐ 600g tempeh (tofu is OK if you can't find any tempeh!)
- ☐ 70g pine nuts (leftover from last week)

- ☐ 50g dessicated coconut
- ☐ 30g sultanas
- ☐ 50g dried cranberries (leftover from week 2)

Fresh herbs

- ☐ Coriander*
- ☐ Mint*
- ☐ Parsley*
- ☐ Dill*
- ☐ Basil

*You may not need to buy these if you have leftovers from previous weeks.

SHOPPING LIST WEEK 4

Dairy alternatives

- [ ] 2 litres soya milk
- [ ] 1 litre hazelnut milk
- [ ] 1 litre almond milk
- [ ] 1 x 255g tub 'Free From' soft cheese

Fruit and vegetables

- [ ] 2 white onions
- [ ] 2 red onions
- [ ] 1 potato (large)
- [ ] 2 sweet potatoes (1 large)
- [ ] 6 spring onions
- [ ] 1 avocado
- [ ] 12 cherry tomatoes
- [ ] 250g baby spinach
- [ ] 2 red peppers
- [ ] 1 bag rocket
- [ ] 18 plum tomatoes
- [ ] 1 small cucumber
- [ ] 150g green beans
- [ ] 1 celeriac
- [ ] 3 carrots
- [ ] 220g chestnut mushrooms
- [ ] 200g wild mushrooms
- [ ] 3 courgettes
- [ ] 300g sundried tomatoes
- [ ] 1 x 280g jar of artichoke hearts
- [ ] 2 limes
- [ ] 5 lemons
- [ ] 350g frozen strawberries
- [ ] 2 pears
- [ ] 8 bananas (put two in the freezer!)
- [ ] 1 small mango
- [ ] 150g dried figs
- [ ] 50g pomegranate seeds
- [ ] 1 x 100g tin pears

Carbohydrate staples

- [ ] 1 pizza base
- [ ] 4 crusty wholemeal rolls
- [ ] 2 vegan naan breads (or flatbreads if you can't find vegan naans)

Dried store foods

- [ ] 1 x 400g tin sweetcorn
- [ ] 1 x 198g tin sweetcorn
- [ ] 200ml coconut milk (leftover from last week)
- [ ] 100g ground almonds
- [ ] 100g silken tofu
- [ ] 2 x 400g tins chickpeas
- [ ] 1 x 400g tin red kidney beans
- [ ] 1 x 400g tin butter beans
- [ ] Dried black lentils
- [ ] 1 x 227g tin chopped tomatoes
- [ ] 100ml coconut cream
- [ ] 250g ready-cooked puy lentils

Other

- [ ] Almond butter
- [ ] 4–6 vegan sausages
- [ ] 130g pine nuts (leftover from week 2)
- [ ] 100g cashews
- [ ] Tamarind paste
- [ ] 70g coconut flakes

Fresh herbs

- [ ] Coriander*
- [ ] Parsley*

*You may not need to buy these if you have leftovers from previous weeks.

SHOPPING LIST WEEK 5

Dairy alternatives
- ☐ 1 x 250g pot of coconut yoghurt
- ☐ 1 litre soya milk

Fruit and vegetables
- ☐ 1 white onion
- ☐ 1 red onion
- ☐ 75g new potatoes
- ☐ 1 sweet potato
- ☐ 2 red peppers
- ☐ 2 tomatoes
- ☐ 8 plum tomatoes
- ☐ 1 aubergine
- ☐ 2 courgettes
- ☐ 4 portobello mushrooms
- ☐ 100g green beans
- ☐ 200g blueberries
- ☐ 2 bananas
- ☐ 4 apricots

Carbohydrate staples
- ☐ Wholemeal bread loaf

Dried store foods
- ☐ 2 x 400ml tins coconut milk

Other
- ☐ 40g massaman curry paste
- ☐ 200g extra-firm tofu
- ☐ 10g dried crushed lavender

Fresh herbs
- ☐ Coriander*
- ☐ Basil*

*You may not need to buy these if there are leftovers from previous weeks.

MENU: WEEK 1

	Breakfast	Lunch	Dinner
Saturday	Mexican brunch bowl	Butternut squash bisque	Savoury oatmeal with sautéed mushrooms and thyme
Sunday	Currant tea loaf with homemade jam	Spiced carrot, date and lentil salad	Chilli non-carne with hummus and avocado
Monday	Mango and coconut smoothie	Sweet potato 'Tex-Mex' salad	Roast vegetable and polenta tart with kale and walnut pesto
Tuesday	Sourdough toast with peanut butter and homemade chia jam	Roasted vegetable and pesto pasta salad	Aromatic crispy tofu stir-fry
Wednesday	Toasted muesli with dried fruit and nuts	Crispy tofu, hummus and avocado pitta	Sweet potato falafel with jewelled couscous
Thursday	Mango and coconut chia pudding	Falafel wrap	Quinoa bowl – baked asparagus, cherry tomatoes, peppers with hummus and balsamic glaze
Friday	Banana, maple syrup and pecan porridge	Mediterranean-inspired sandwiches	Linguine with a mushroom and chestnut sauce

MENU: WEEK 2

	Breakfast	Lunch	Dinner
Saturday	Quinoa granola with dried raspberries and cacao nibs	Broad bean, asparagus and mint tartine	A Lebanese feast: Imam, hummus, flatbread and a nutty kale salad
Sunday	Pancakes with stewed autumn fruits and coconut yoghurt	Fennel and white bean soup	Caponata-inspired spaghetti
Monday	Chia pudding with coconut, pomegranate and pistachios	Artichoke and broad bean salad with a tahini dressing	Red Thai butter bean curry with wild rice
Tuesday	Berry blast smoothie	Rainbow wild rice salad with a tangy dressing	Korean quinoa bowls
Wednesday	Multi-grain porridge	Nutty quinoa salad with fresh veggies and mustard vinaigrette	'Shepherd-less' pie with sweet potato mash
Thursday	Smashed avocado and spiced chickpeas on toast	Fennel, white bean and courgetti salad with tahini dressing	Beetroot sliders
Friday	Apricot, blueberry and hazelnut bircher muesli	Leftover beetroot sliders with buckwheat tabbouleh	Lemon and pea risotto with roasted asparagus spears

MENU: WEEK 3

	Breakfast	Lunch	Dinner
Saturday	Raw date, pecan and walnut breakfast bars	Borscht	Aubergine katsu curry
Sunday	Rösti topped with rocket and mashed avo	Hot aubergine pockets	Tempeh kebabs with a peanut dipping sauce
Monday	Layered summer fruit parfait with coconut yoghurt and granola	Sourdough fattoush with butter beans	Sweet potato and chickpea curry with a spiced tomato salad
Tuesday	Cacao, date and banana smoothie	Indian-spiced tomato and white bean salad	Quinoa bowl – harissa roasted aubergine, garlic mushrooms, spinach and hummus
Wednesday	Apple and ginger bircher muesli	Gado-gado with quinoa	Vegan quinoa sushi
Thursday	Tropical popical smoothie	Mango, tomato and basil salad	Spinach crepes with a pepper filling
Friday	Porridge with vanilla poached plums	Turkish tomato salad with coconut haydari	Quinoa-stuffed peppers with Moroccan flavours

MENU: WEEK 4

	Breakfast	Lunch	Dinner
Saturday	Banana, fig and pear muffins	Raw carrot gazpacho	Vegan sausages with truffle mash
Sunday	Spicy sweetcorn fritters with avocado and coriander	Toasted spiced chickpea salad	Vegan pizzas with roasted tomato hummus
Monday	Strawberry and soya breakfast smoothie	Sweetcorn and bean wrap	Coconut and tamarind curry
Tuesday	Pear and date bircher muesli	Hummus and grilled courgette wrap	Mushroom and rocket polenta tart with gremolata
Wednesday	Almond butter, pomegranate and fig	Lentil salad with gremolata	Spaghetti with a creamy artichoke sauce
Thursday	Berry and vanilla chia pudding with a crunchy granola topping	Tartine with artichoke paté and pan-fried vegetables	Coconut and tomato daal with a zesty mango salad
Friday	Peanut butter and frozen banana smoothie	Quinoa mango salad	'Beany' chow

MENU: WEEK 5

	Breakfast	Lunch	Dinner
Saturday	Vegan French toast 'pockets' with blueberries and cinnamon	Sweet potato, corn and coconut soup	Ratatouille-stuffed mushrooms with a pearl barley salad
Sunday	Pancakes with apricots, lavender, coconut yoghurt and agave	Sourdough bruschetta	Tofu massaman curry